JOURNEY THROUGH ALZHEIMER'S

COMPASSIONATE CAREGIVING

B. Geraldine Meggait

Order this book online at www.trafford.com
or email orders@trafford.com

Most Trafford titles are also available at major online book retailers.

Print information available on the last page.

ISBN: 978-1-4120-4431-8 (sc)
ISBN: 978-1-4907-5544-1 (e)

Trafford rev. 02/10/2015

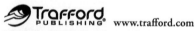 www.trafford.com

North America & international
toll-free: 1 888 232 4444 (USA & Canada)
fax: 812 355 4082

**DEDICATED
TO THE MEMORY OF MY MOTHER,
VERTA POUNCY**

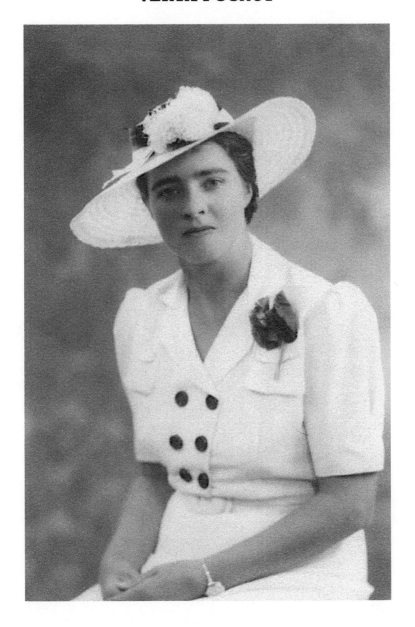

A GRACIOUS LADY

My Mother: A Gracious Lady

Mother's hands were gentle. Her words were kind and caring. She was as close to pure love as is possible to find in this world. She had four children. I was the oldest then in order came Joyce, Faith Alica, and Frank. She rarely had to correct us, because her unconditional love was so great that we had no desire to do wrong. When she did correct us, it was with love and gentleness. I'll never forget Mom's hands soothing our fevered foreheads. Her love was totally encompassing. Even during the last few days, she kept telling me how much she loved me; but not only me, she loved each one of her children, grandchildren, great grandchildren, and indeed the children and people of the world. To me she epitomized love.

ACKNOWLEDGEMENTS

Special thanks to:

* ❀ My siblings and each one of my precious family for support, encouragement, and help with editing.
* ❀ The Armstrong Home Support Staff.
* ❀ Donna MacNaughton and other caregivers who helped to support my mother and enhance her life.
* ❀ All those who gave my mother care in her illness— particularly Drs. Clement and Sherwin, the pharmacists at Armstrong Pharmacy & Wellness Centre, the surgeon and nurses who gave mother such loving care during her last illness in Vernon Jubilee Hospital.
* ❀ Twyla Proud, RN, whose encouragement was invaluable to me.
* ❀ Lois Mollard for the artistry of the cover design.
* ❀ Shirley Campbell for her willingness to share her knowledge of the writing process.

Thanks also to:

* ❀ All those who taught me throughout my life that gentleness, respect, kindness, and love were all worthwhile personal goals.
* ❀ My friends and supporters at Kindale Developmental Association, and First Baptist Church, Armstrong, BC

Table Of Contents

INTRODUCTION

The purpose of this book is simply to help others who are traveling through the same vicious journey that my mother and I traveled.

It is not my intention to give professional or medical opinions, but just to relay my experiences. As I journeyed with my mother through the disease, I came to some conclusions. These may, or may not, apply to other people.

The stories in the book are not written chronologically. Although that might have been helpful to readers, it was hard for me to remember occurrences in sequence. Most of the excerpts from my journal were written in the last two years of my mother's life.

My intent is to have a warm, personal book because that's who mother was and who I ever hope to be. The stories are personal and emotional; because of that I wrote slowly and took frequent breaks. My desire is that even the stories convey the viciousness of the disease, and even more importantly, the worth of a human being. Even such a dreadful disease as Alzheimer's cannot erase every vestige of the precious human being and we should never forget that. Though the loved one may forget your face and your name, she can know the gentle touch of your hand and the heart-warming smile on your face. She can fully experience the love of your heart. Your situation may be much different from mine, but you can make a difference! I did!

PART ONE

BEGINNINGS

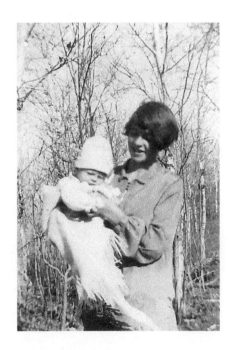

Verta Pouncy
with the author as baby, 1928

1. OH, SO SLOWLY

It started oh, so slowly. First I noticed that Mom was concerned about her memory. She wanted to take a course that would help it. In her eighties, I thought that she was just growing old and it was a normal part of aging. I was so very wrong; there was nothing normal about the memory loss that my mother was experiencing. Still I did not recognize it for what it really was. She had begun a journey that was slow but inevitable, and from which she could not escape. Mother started to get mixed up on the days of the week. Most troubling to her was the perceived loss of her precious jewelry. She was living in a secured seniors housing apartment complex and her doors were locked every night. I could not figure out how it was possible for someone to come in and steal it without her knowledge. Then she reported that her government pension cheque did not arrive in the mail. The bills started piling up. She was receiving junk-jewelry in the mail and sending money for it. I finally realized that my wonderful mother simply could not remember. From that time on, my son Tony or I supervised her mail and the payment of her bills.

One day a cousin from England was visiting Mother in her apartment when she received a phone call from someone who said she had won a new car. They asked her to send some money so they could deliver it. Of course he recognized it was a scam and reported it to us. Somehow her name had been put on a "sucker list" and she was paying good money for nothing. When our cousin told me, Mom was annoyed: "I wanted to surprise you when I received my new car."

Just a few days ago, I was destroying some of Mom's

old, useless business papers when I came across two months of canceled cheques. There were hundreds of dollars' worth of cheques made out to bogus companies. In disgust I burned them all. What moral depravity to prey on the elderly and infirm! I don't understand such self-centered behavior.

My son Gordie's wife, Karen, had noticed Mom's memory loss more than ten years before the disease became manifest to most of us. She noticed that Mom could not remember her address although she could still find her way home from the store, and from the hospital where she had been visiting my Dad.

This was the very beginning. Still later in the disease I noticed that Mom could not remember the names of common, familiar everyday items, or the names of various family members. I had heard of a condition called anomia and thought that described her problems. Although she always retained the ability to communicate at an elemental level, she coped by using general words. She became quite adept at covering up her disabilities—a loving smile went a long way. If people greeted her warmly she greeted them warmly in return. Casual acquaintances had little concept of the severity of her disease.

2. A THUMBNAIL SKETCH OF HER LIFE

Mother was born to a father of Irish descent who left an indelible mark on her personality. Although I have never been able to verify her story, Mother told me that he was born on a ship coming over from Ireland. Influenced by her Irish heritage, Mom loved laughter, people, and God.

She had music and rhythm coming out of the tips of her toes. From her mother of English descent she learned caring and responsibility, cooking for threshing gangs (when she was only twelve) and looking after the many children that joined their family.

In 1926 she eloped and married my father—a handsome gentleman who had emigrated from England. She was not yet eighteen. Mom and Dad went into farming. While cutting some logs in a small mill, Dad accidentally slipped on some ice and fell into the saw. That put an end to his ability to work for a year or two—back in the 'dirty thirties' it was quite a job for him simply to stay alive. They decided to move into the little Manitoban village about six miles away. As Dad slowly became better he decided that somehow he must make some money to support the family. My father was a brilliant man with many natural abilities. He converted a two-car garage into a service station and made an agreement with an oil company to get him started in business. So he was set up. Mom was fully his working partner in all the future business enterprises in which he became involved: garages, grocery stores, general merchandise stores, etc. Her capabilities and flexibility always showed.

Besides her business ventures with Dad, mother quilted, cooked, sewed, gardened, wallpapered, painted (oils, pastels, textile and china) and created many various kinds of crafts. She was always busy and purposeful. The local doctor often called her to assist him delivering babies, and performing tonsillectomies. She even drove a taxi. Mom had multi-interests and multi-talents.

In 1947 they moved to Vernon, British Columbia, and later to nearby Armstrong—both in the beautiful Okanagan Valley. My Dad had always yearned for a warmer climate than that of Manitoba. They continued operating businesses until they decided to semi-retire. Still active they farmed, tended a golf course, and even worked one winter at a ski hill. For some time, Mom helped my sister, Alica, in a Kindergarten class. Mother had an inner and outer beauty. Her belief in God and spiritual matters were very real and important to her and gave her purpose and zeal.

It was to this very beautiful person that this dreadful disease occurred. We cannot rationalize why terrible things sometimes happen to good people. We can only say that problems are a part of the human condition and none of us are exempt.

3. RETIREMENT

In the early 1980s, Dad was diagnosed with Parkinson's disease and that ended their working careers. In 1981, Mom could no longer care for him and he was hospitalized. Mom was faithful in visiting every day. She continued to live in the condominium that they had shared. As the years stretched on, the family became concerned about her health. Then as now, we lived on a farm outside of Armstrong and we encouraged her to purchase and live in a house across from us. She did as we wished, and that enabled us to help her. Dad's life ended in 1988. Mother enjoyed her home and garden, but soon after Dad died she was forced to sell her home because of declining health. She moved into a rented apartment in a facility for seniors, just four miles from our home right in Armstrong.

4. MOTHER'S LAST HOME

My sister, Alica, and her husband Richard, holiday annually in Hawaii. Mother joined them for a week each year. She loved this vacation. We would take her to the

Kelowna Airport about fifty miles away and leave her with the personnel. In Vancouver my sister and her husband always met her. This method worked well for a number of years. Gradually we began to realize that things were not perfect. One time Mom came home and said that she had been unable to wash her hands all the time she was away because she couldn't operate the faucets. On a flight home from visiting another daughter who lived in Manitoba, she said she was in agony while on the plane. She did not know where to locate the washroom, and did not understand that she should ask the flight attendant

One day my son, Tony, met Mom at the airport. Before coming home she used the washroom in the terminal. Because of her diminished comprehension she was unable to find her way out of the washroom. Poor Mom—life was beginning to close in on her.

When she returned from her last trip, she became very ill. I said, "Mom, would you like to stay with us for a few days?" She said, "Yes." By the end of the week, she was feeling better and we were expecting overnight guests. Mom said, *"I guess I have to go home."* Immediately I picked up on her reluctance to leave. I said, "Mom, would you like to come and live with us?" She simply said, *"Yes."*

So, my very independent mother came to live with us. Something she had vowed never to do. Earlier I had been so worried. How were we ever to move her? How would she adjust to the loss of her independence? Yet in the end it had been so easy. When my beloved mother came to live with us, it marked the beginning of a very special phase in my life. Yes, there were hard times ahead—much worry and much fear, but precious nevertheless.

5. MAKING IT POSSIBLE

Some people have elaborate plans in the event that they cannot care for themselves. More often, it comes suddenly: a fall, an illness, a death in the family, or some other traumatic occurrence. Suddenly you encounter an emergency. There may be no openings in the medical system for your loved one, or you may truly want to be the primary caregiver—yet your life is full. How is it possible to take on this additional burden?

For Martin and me, we had long ago assumed a great deal of responsibility for both sets of parents. This is primarily because of location—we lived near them. For most of our married lives we had been caring for someone: our children, foster children, a man with disabilities, and the list goes on and on. So we were not strangers to caregiving.

My dad was the first parent who needed care. He had Parkinson's disease for a number of years, and for the last six and one half years of his life he was hospitalized. I had a great desire to care for him but he was six feet tall and immobile, and rightly or wrongly I thought I was unable to care for him in our home. I was able to visit him often in the Extended Care wing of the hospital though, and I was with him when he died.

The next parent was Martin's mother. At almost 95 years of age, she fell and broke her pelvis and came to live with us. She had been living independently in town with minimal support. Suddenly everything changed—she needed help and right now. I was at the height of my career as a Manager of Programming at a developmental center for persons with disabilities, and I did not want to quit my job. Somehow I had to achieve quality care without my personal attendance twenty-four hours a day. We took advantage of government Home Support to help us. In addition, we took the money that would have been used for board and room, and some small savings she had, and hired reliable companions to assist her. Of course, Martin and I cared for her evenings, nights and holidays. This seemed to work well for the two and one half years that she lived with us.

Lastly, Mother needed care. I was still working and my job was absolutely important in my life, and so was caring for my mother in a loving and beneficial way. We had the same sort of arrangement as we had for my mother-in-law—the money that she had been using to run her apartment and for food, etc., we now used for personal care. We were also privileged to have the support of Home Care. There was a small cost to us. In addition to some personal financial outlay for Mother, there were also some costs related to the caregivers in daily attendance; however, it was within our budget and no burden to us.

WHERE THERE'S A WILL THERE'S A WAY

- a frequent quote by my mother

PART TWO

THE DISEASE
AND
ADAPTATIONS
TO IT

1. MEMORY LOSS

One of the outstanding characteristics of Alzheimer's disease is that there is no permanent solution to any problem. At first solutions might work for a month at a time, then for a week, and towards the end changes might have to be done daily. Flexibility is extremely important, and solving problems is constant.

Foundational to all the problems was the loss of memory. Several times a day, mother went into the washroom and her bedroom. Occasionally she viewed them with wonder, as in this occasion when she went to the washroom and excitedly said, *"Oh, here's a room I've never been in. I'm going in to see it!"* The same happened a few times when she went into her bedroom: *"Isn't this nice!"* Even though she didn't really remember, it seemed to offer her comfort. The same happened with the wicker chair that had been my mother-in-law's, and the big chair in the living room. More often her emotion was confusion and fear.

To illustrate the memory loss, the following are some excerpts from my journal:

October 28, 1997: Physical (examination) took one and one-half hours. Mom was in a housecoat and had lots of procedures done. When Martin came in soon after, he asked her if she had seen the doctor. She said, "No". (No memory of it left.)

December 28, 1997: Mom had quite a bit of confusion last night: "What do I do with this (her drink)? What do I do with this (her crackers)?" I'm glad she can communicate verbally and with signs. It helps me know what is bothering her. Mother cranky: "I don't know anything. I don't know my own name." Got her off to bed. Tried to lighten her mood.

January 16, 1998: Yesterday Mother picked up an envelope that I had received from my friend Lena in

Ochre River. She tried to read 'Ochre River' and stumbled over it. I said, "Ochre River—do you remember Ochre River?" She responded "No." I replied, "You lived there for a long time." With resignation she responded, "Good." It is hard to fathom such complete loss of a large part of her life, and almost all our childhood.

January 17, 1998: The other night I gave her four buttered crackers and warm water. She ate the crackers. I immediately asked her if she wanted some more crackers. She answered, "Oh, I haven't had any."

January 24, 1998: 8 p.m. Mom said, "I can't remember anything. Where am I?" I told her who she was, about Dad and his death, coming to our place, her room and bed. Mom: "I have a bed here? Well, who am I?" Then she asked a second time, "Who am I?" I told her. She said, "What is wrong with me that I can't remember?" I replied, "You have a sickness that takes the memories away." I told her the memories are there it's just hard to get them out. I said, "You remember your Dad—the big man?" She responded, "Yes, and I remember my mother too. I saw my mother yesterday. When will I see my mother again?" Me: "I'm not sure. Sometimes when you're not expecting her she will be here." (It is useless to tell her that her mother is dead, as she believes her mother is here at times.) We talked some more and she asked again where she was. "What is this place? Who is he (indicating Martin)?" Although she didn't ask who I was, I told her. Mom sighed a lot and said, "Oh dear." Then she asked how old she was. When I told her she replied with amazement, "Eighty-nine!"

Strangely enough, occasionally she would have a little sliver of memory break through. On October 31, 1997, mother amazed everyone when she reminded our son Tony of the time about fifteen years previously when she and Tony had danced together at a Hallowe'en Party.

There were daily incidences of sad memory losses,

and this book will reveal many of them. Memory loss is an essential characteristic of the disease and tends to result in confusion, paranoia, depression, and sometimes aggression.

Another illustration of a memory loss took place on November 28, 1997: *Mom seems a little better (physically) but has slipped mentally. The Home Support worker said that last night she lifted her cup partway to her mouth to drink tea, then hesitated not remembering whether she was raising or lowering the cup.*

2. DISCOURAGEMENT AND DEPRESSION

Mother constantly battled discouragement. Her loss of memory produced confusion. Everything was very disturbing to her. Along with the discouragement came depression. We constantly worked to help her overcome both.

August 8, 1997: (Mom) talking a bit depressed. "I'm not dead yet. It wouldn't matter if I fell and died." Her confusion is acute. January 13, 1998: Wouldn't eat supper—too tired. Bed (slept) till 6:45 p.m. Offered supper. Refused—too tired. Sitting in front room now. She said, "I'm just too tired." Put her to bed 7:10. She said, "I'm just so tired. I hope I don't wake up."

Amazingly, Mother sometimes bounced back. She was a very resilient person. Despite her resilience, serious memory loss and confusion inevitably led to discouragement and depression. I believe you will find this truth revealed throughout my book. My writing will also reveal some of the techniques we used to alleviate the situation—it was not possible to completely remedy it.

3. FEAR AND AGITATION

Fears surrounded my mother daily, particularly as the evening fell, and during the night. The evening was frightening for many reasons: tiredness, reflections, darkness, and the ever-present lack of memory. Night was frightening because every time she awoke, she thought she was in a strange place, with strangers tending to her. (She often did not recognize Martin or me when she first woke up.) Of course, thunderstorms were especially frightening.

Sometimes even visiting family members, whom she often recognized, were feared. The following is an excerpt from my journal written by one of her Home Support workers:

August 21, 1996: Verta very distraught at "Strangers" in the living room (two grandchildren and one friend— teens). Wished Gerry would tell them to get out. Stayed agitated until she thought she heard them leave. I had to do considerable distracting, etc. Stayed close as Verta became shaky.

4. EATING

Adaptations to Eating

Just as in every area of the disease, mother's ability and interest in eating varied, and we had to make frequent adaptations.

In the beginning she ate quite normally. Slowly she lost the ability to discern how much she had eaten or how recently. If she saw someone eating, she thought that she must eat as well—even if she saw food sitting on a table or counter, then she thought she was hungry. She lost all sense of hunger and satiety.

A couple of years before her death, she had a bout

of pneumonia. She was very ill. After she came home from the hospital, she refused to eat all solids. I pureed all her food and made soup for each meal. After a time, perhaps some weeks, mother became tired of soup, so slowly I introduced soft foods back into her diet. In the latter years she never was able to tolerate certain solids or roughage.

The other caregivers and I kept a food diary for Mother. Just as in all areas there were significant daily changes in the manner in which she responded to food. Food was presented at regular meal times and whenever she requested it. Although she wanted to eat when it wasn't mealtime, she might only take a bite or two. Overeating and excess weight were not problems for Mom. Getting some nutrition into her, and keeping her happy and contented were priorities. That might not be the case with some other people.

Mother liked small bits of food she could pick up in her fingers; such as, French Fries and Chicken Chunks. For a treat we sometimes took her out to a fast food restaurant. I think it was the softness and ease of handling that she liked.

Towards the end of her life, she once again refused foods. Sometimes she was just too tired to eat or drink, other times she did not know what food and drink were. *"What am I supposed to do with this?"* she would say with confusion and sometimes disgust. We tried our very best to present her with foods that she liked in ways that were most appealing. We gave her a small plate. Each different food would be arranged on the plate separately from each other and in small amounts. At times she refused to eat; at other times she would possibly eat crackers, small amounts of mashed potatoes, squash, perhaps a wee piece of ham or soft chicken, bananas, Rice Crispy squares, and small amounts of toast or bread. If something did not please her, she would push it away.

Sometimes she did weird things with her food. One day we had given her some food on a plate as usual. She took her cup of tea and poured it over her food, and then mixed it up. We made no comment, and treated it like it was an ordinary event—this allowed Mom to retain her dignity. This was far more important than whether or not she mixed tea in with her food. Mother was past learning new things and we recognized that.

Martin supervised her breakfast while I slept for a little longer. He often served her on a TV tray at a wicker chair raised with a foam pad, and that had arms to help her sit down and rise up more easily. Towards the end of her life when our family came for dinner, I would sit with Mom in another room to eat. That was because the noise and activity confused my mother too much. She did better with quietness and peace, even though it was important for the family to get together. Earlier in the disease, she would often rise to the occasion and try to be the hostess and entertain people—often showing particular concern for someone she perceived as older than she was.

During her final days in the hospital, the nutritionist tried to encourage her appetite. The surgeon told us that if she would just eat and drink she would live. All efforts were useless. Mother gave up although we tried to give her small amounts of yogurt. In the end her dementia, rather than her broken hip, caused her death. She did not seem to recognize food or how important it was to sustain life.

January 30, 1998: Didn't really eat well. I sat her at the table with a mid-sized plate instead of in her own chair with the food on a bread and butter plate. I'm always worried about inclusion, but it seemed too confusing and overwhelming—I'll go back to my usual.

Varied Eating Problems

The problems that assailed my mother during the final years of her life were many and varied. One day she tried to eat her diamond ring. Another day she pointed to a flower that decorated her TV tray and said, *"Do I eat this?"* I traded that tray for one that was plain brown and undecorated.

Sometimes Mom had a very subtle way of saying she wanted to eat, although I am sure she was not capable of intentional subtlety. One day I was cleaning the living room. She had eaten recently when she said to me: *"When are we going to eat?"* I patiently explained that she had eaten just a little while ago, and I wanted to finish cleaning and then I would get lunch. *"OK,"* she said. I started cleaning again. Almost immediately she pointed to Martin's picture and said, *"He wants to eat."* At that I went and got her a couple of buttered graham wafers—that made her happy.

One of the problems I experienced was that my husband and son ate lunch at different times from the rest of us. If mother saw anyone eating she had to eat too, or she thought she was being denied food and became very angry. We coped with these various problems by giving her small amounts of food whenever she showed an interest in eating. I realize that in a group or hospital setting this is not always possible, but I also realize that if we had not done this, we would have encountered much agitation, anger, and aggression.

Some of her problems were comical, and left me not knowing whether to laugh or cry—they were both sad and funny. Of course to her they were very serious and disturbing. Sometimes she dipped her slice of cooked carrot in her tea or into a slice of potato.

Eating Variations in the Day

Mother ate food much better in the morning. As the day progressed, problems tended to gain in significance. Here is an excerpt from my journal:

January 13, 1998 (less than two months before she died): By night, I hardly think she knows what her food and drinks are. It wasn't long ago that she was eating carrots, squash, and mashed potatoes—now turning them all down. Her favourites—pancakes and baking powder biscuits—she'll take earlier in the day. By supper nothing seems to tempt her to eat. After a sleep, usually about 8 p.m., she eats three or four buttered crackers. Her diet is heavy to bread and crackers, but I can't help it.

February 11, 1998, 4:30 p.m.: Mom wanted to eat—said it smelled good. Gave her a saucer of mashed baked potato and squash. She ate a couple of spoonfuls and started to divide it up for the 'others'. I told her I had lots of food for others—but it didn't help, so I took it away. I told her she looked tired, but she said (immediately after turning away the food): "I'm waiting around for other things to eat. That's all I care about 'things to eat'." At 5:30 p.m.: Gave her a little turnip and macaroni; ate very little (a bite or two given to her on a bread and butter plate). She seemed very confused and dependent; pointing to different foods: "What shall I do with this—or this—or this?" 6 p.m. Put her to bed.

Dreaming about Food

Sometimes it seemed that my mother must have been dreaming about food, because her statements had no basis in fact. Here is one taken from my journal:

Mom told me that she had worked and worked to prepare food—a whole lot of it. Then someone came in and took it all. The person never gave her, or anyone else, any of it. She whispered, "Don't say anything to anybody." She held the story in her mind for a couple of hours and retold it. I assured her we had lots of food and I would get her anything she wanted.

5. DINING OUT

Mother loved to go and do—whatever the activity. Often we took her out for Sunday lunch.

One Sunday, we took her to a restaurant with a great smorgasbord. We chose many of the wonderful options for her, and she ate with great gusto. After we were all finished, I said to Mom, "Well Mom, how did you enjoy that lunch?" Seriously she responded, *"Well, it wasn't the worst lunch I've ever had, but it was close to it!"* Despite her obvious enjoyment, her memory was so short-lived that she had already forgotten. Of course, I was quietly amused.

It was important to ensure that Mom's behaviour was appropriate in public. I remember once that she took the ends of her scarf and used it for a napkin. We were always gentle and redirected her to the best of our abilities.

Even though my mother loved going into the community and eating at various restaurants, sometimes these outings also caused confusion. It was on Tony's birthday, November 30, 1997, that we took her to his party at a restaurant. She was angry and upset, we didn't know why. Karen and the girls (our son Gordie's wife and children) tried to get her on track, but couldn't. She was upset about the serviette. She said it wasn't hers, but when I tried to remove it she became protective and irritated. We all had to wait while they prepared the food. Mother became angrier because she thought there was nothing to eat. I asked for some crackers and she ate them while we waited for our dinners. She remained feisty even when we arrived home. I thought perhaps she was overtired. It was hard to know whether or not it best to exclude her from family celebrations because sometimes she really enjoyed them.

6. CONVERSATIONS

Although Mom was able to express her ideas very simply, conversations were difficult. She did not have the ability to understand or respond appropriately. It was particularly disturbing to her when she overheard conversations that were not geared to her level of comprehension.

One day Martin was angrily presenting his views on a serial child killer. Mom misunderstood and complained to me, *"Your man is looking at me. He thinks I am stupid."* Of course the conversation had nothing whatever to do with her.

I recorded in my journal that I could hardly talk to Martin because she constantly questioned and misinterpreted everything that we said. Of course that made daily life quite difficult and I had to work hard to dispel her confusion.

7. TAKING MEDICATIONS

Sometimes Mother took her medications without objection, while at other times she adamantly refused them. Usually, her mind was clearer in the morning and so there was more compliance then.

Our method for presenting her pills was to ask her to take them, and watch that she swallowed them (she liked to tuck them into a Kleenex or into her pocket). One time she was heard to say, *"I'll just save these for the children."* So constant vigilance was vitally important.

If she refused, we did not coax or insist, we just quietly removed them. We kept on presenting them again and again at five-minute intervals until she finally took them. Of course, because of her memory loss she did not remember that she had refused them previously. Occasionally, we were unable to get her to take them at all.

January 11, 1997: First fight of my life with Mom on Thursday night. She refused meds, put them in a Kleenex and carried them off. I traded a new Kleenex for the one with pills. She became extremely angry. I said, "Mom, I don't want to cross you but if the children get hold of those pills, they could kill them." She just became angrier. I just took the pills and threw them in the garbage—then I busied myself around in the kitchen. Before long she had forgotten—must watch pills at all times.

In retrospect, I might have avoided the argument if I had said something like the following: "Mom, why don't we find a pretty dish to put your pills in. Later you can have them if you wish." That would most likely have been a satisfactory solution to Mother. To suggest that she would (as she might interpret my actual response) ever intentionally harm a child would certainly have angered her.

The following is a list of instructions about medications given to caregivers who came into our home:

May 1997: Presenting Pills: Always watch. She may drop pills on floor, roll in Kleenexes, put up sleeve, put in Kleenex box, put in food/drink, etc. Usually (she) takes pills OK in morning but as day wears on, she tires, and sometimes refuses pills. If she isn't overly confused I offer again. If very confused, I accept her refusal as her choice. At supper I usually offer Serc first (to prevent Meniere's attack and vomiting). At night, I offer Oxazapam first as it is a mild tranquilizer. If she is extremely agitated the doctor said she could be given a whole Oxazapam. (I haven't given a whole one yet.)

8. MOTHER'S DRIVING

While Mom was still living by herself in the apartment, the complaints started to come to me. Mom couldn't find her apartment. Mother had trouble finding the ignition to start her car and her driving was erratic. She should not be driving. I knew how important it was for her. She loved to give rides to the other seniors in the complex. It represented two things: her independence, and her ability to help others—something she had always done. I waited for someone to take responsibility—her doctor or the Motor Vehicle Branch. No one did. Finally, I realized I had to act; no one else was doing it. Of course I should have explained the situation to her doctor and asked for specific intervention. I failed to do this.

Mother sat on the chair stoically as I talked to her. Her face was a mask. I started by saying, "Mom, remember when you had to tell Dad he shouldn't drive anymore? Well, now I have to tell you. You have helped people all your life; wouldn't it be a tragedy if you hit or killed someone? You mustn't drive anymore."

Tears silently rolled down my mother's cheeks. Still she did not say anything. About forty-five minutes later she finally spoke, *"Well, I may as well die. There is nothing left for me." Love mixed with responsibility can be very difficult at times. I had to hurt the very person I loved so much!*

For the rest of her life mother periodically grieved over the loss of her driving independence. "Someone told me I couldn't drive anymore," she would say in sorrow and sometimes in anger. Fortunately for me she forgot that I was the one who had told her.

Soon after that, Mom came to live with Martin and me. She still owned her car, and the woman hired to enhance her life drove her to activities; such as, seniors' luncheons, craft parties, sing-songs, or just out for lunch or tea. Mother loved activity and people, and these activities greatly enriched her life. Mom agreed to pay for the gas and any costs incurred by the activities.

9. ACTIVITIES

Planned activities for mother are woven throughout all my writing. Mom had always been very active. Painting in various forms had been one of her passions. I recall one day she wanted to try to do some china painting after not doing it for some time. She shut herself in the bedroom. After an hour or two of failed attempts she came out and never tried again.

At first when she came to live with us there were simple jobs that she was able to do: folding towels and washing a few dishes. (I put them in the dishwasher after, for sanitary purposes. She never understood the function of the dishwasher.) Her companion did some very simple crafts with her. As time went by, she could do none of these things and it became very difficult to keep her busy and contented. As her disease progressed, Mother began to do things compulsively: folding napkins, Kleenexes, and toilet paper. She was obsessively neat and tidy.

Mother liked music, and I would put on a tape of lively Irish music, or I would play the piano in my amateurish fashion. She also liked batting balloons. She did not react well to TV, or too much noise and confusion—she seemed to adapt better to the quiet life. Of course, she liked car rides, going for pie and coffee, and meeting people.

Quite early in the disease we drove to Manitoba from BC, and took Mother with us. Her memory was starting to deteriorate and confusion was beginning. We stayed one night at a motel. We were able to book adjoining rooms and I left the door unlocked between the two. I settled Mother for the night and left a note written in large letters: GERRY IS IN THE NEXT ROOM. SHE WILL CALL YOU IN THE MORNING. Fortunately, all went well. Although she loved traveling, that was the last long trip we made with her.

One day when Mom and I were alone, I took her out into the yard and wrapped her up warmly (she always seemed to be cold). She watched me as I watered plants and dug up a little flowerbed. Nearby the cats frolicked and birds flittered about. Mother thoroughly enjoyed that time and it had a relaxing effect.

Prior to living with us she loved to bake. We always enjoyed her pies, especially lemon ones. She also made excellent buns and biscuits. When we moved her, we found multiple bowls with partially mixed ingredients for baking powder biscuits. Although we knew she was losing memory, we truly did not realize how far the disease had progressed.

One of the things Mother loved to do was to go to church. Martin and I took her out to church until near the very end of her life. She seemed to receive some comfort from going. She was in a friendly environment—everyone loved her and demonstrated it. She loved the old hymns and gentle words. In the later stages of the disease, I debated about taking her for Communion Sunday, which was once a month. I did not think she understood. I feared that if I did not allow her to take the cracker and juice, she would think she was being denied; however if she did, she might spill the grape juice. Sometimes, we were able to quietly pass the juice without her noticing it.

The following excerpts from my journal describe some of the difficulties we had in choosing suitable activities:

August 16, 1997: Mom likes my playing a little, but has very little interests—hard to entertain. One of the problems is that as soon as an event is past she forgets that it ever happened—so life is boring.

September 21, 1997: Yesterday Mom was restful until about 2:30 p.m., and then nothing settled her. I gave her the special book I had prepared for her. "That's it," she said definitely and shut the book. I gave her a book of pretty cards, "But what can I do with this?" and she'd point to the picture of a flower. She kept on obsessing on all the flowers in the same manner until I put the book away—the same happened with pictures of babies. Then she wanted to gather up things to go—to take with her. When I asked where she was going, she said, "I don't know". Finally in desperation I took her out to pick the last of the fall flowers. Wintertime is to come and how to redirect is a real serious consideration. I took her out to supper at a local restaurant just for a change. It is expensive to do it too often.

January 31, 1998: Mom is very puzzled over a book about mothers that I gave her. I put her name in it and she goes over and over the fact that it mentions her name. I pointed out several times that it says, "Love, Gerry", but most of the time she doesn't recognize me as Gerry. She often enjoys looking at books with many pictures, even children's books. She particularly enjoyed the children's book, "Who is my mother?" She was always searching for her identity.

10. MONEY

As time went on Mom started to forget that she had agreed to financial arrangements and she complained, *"Why do I always have to pay for everything?"*

Money became a serious problem. Fortunately she had given my son, Tony, signing authority on all her financial accounts and he was able to write cheques to cover her obligations—which to us were not numerous but to her became a major issue.

The only time I remember momentarily becoming a little angry with my mother was over the payment of her medical coverage. As I usually did, I wrote out a cheque and gave it to her to sign. Angrily she refused to sign it. Against my better judgment I tried to reason with her. She had always signed cheques without questions She was adamant in her refusal. I felt a combination of frustration and anger. I walked away from her through the hall, living room, dining room, and back to the kitchen where she was still standing. By then I was totally composed and at peace with her lack of understanding, and from then on money dealings were done through Tony. This was a great convenience to us.

Money held a great importance to Mom. Dad had always controlled the finances and when he died, she finally had the ability to make financial decisions. We always ensured that she had spending money in her purse so that she could maintain her sense of financial independence.

11. CLOTHING

An Elegant Lady

Yesterday, more than six years after her death, a woman said to me, "I remember your mother so well.

She was so kind and caring. She was an elegant lady." I thought, 'How well that describes my Mom. She was elegant'. Even in her younger years she never wore slacks unless she was gardening or selling tickets on the ski hill. She always dressed with style, and held herself in a queen-like manner. In many ways she was like the queen mother, Elizabeth—royal in every way.

Mom went to the hairdresser every week, and while never vain took an interest in how she appeared. She and her hairdresser had a very special relationship for many years. He was very good to her.

I was always amazed at how mother never seemed to get dirty. She had a knack for looking elegant even when doing the messiest work.

Changing Abilities

At first Mom was capable of choosing her own clothing and dressing herself. When she started wearing some very strange combinations, we began to lay out her clothing at night for the next morning. We had to close her closet door so she wouldn't try to dress herself. Once it was closed she did not seem to recognize that her clothes were in it. Later it was a matter of leaving only her housecoat out, and a Home Care worker would come in, give her a bath, and dress her. It was a matter of frequent adaptations to her changing functioning abilities.

Fashionable Still

One day I was discussing Mom's condition with her doctor. "One thing about my mother is that she has never lost her sense of fashion."

"Oh," replied the doctor, "does she dress herself?"

I kept remembering this conversation after I left the doctor's office. No, she didn't dress herself. She had a great deal of help. But there was always something about her choice of clothing and the way she carried herself that gave me the knowledge that mother still had a sense of fashion. It might also have been that when she saw me dressed up especially nicely, she commented on how well I looked. Her remarks about clothing and fashion always seemed appropriate.

One day Mom dressed herself. She was able to get on all her clothing. The last thing she put on was her slip. It was beautiful—silky and covered with lace. Not actually appropriate but in another society it might be classy!

The Ugly Slippers

When Mom came to live with us, she had some pastel blue slippers. She really liked her slippers. Because of her problems with diarrhea the slippers had to be washed frequently. Soon they became useless and broken down. I went to various stores looking for new slippers—preferably just like them. I could not find any.

I chose a pair of blue slippers. They looked comfortable. I thought Mother would really like them as she was constantly cold and they were warm. Instantly Mom took a dislike to them. *"Whoever would wear these?"* she complained. "Oh, Mom, they are so warm. They will keep your feet so nice and cozy." At hearing my words, Mother screwed up her face with disgust and said, *"Oh yes, they are warm, but they are so ugly."*

One of Mom's companions brought a couple of bright shiny decorations and sewed them on the sides—indicating left and right feet. Although Mother wore them it was reluctantly, and she often said, *"Oh, these are so ugly. Whoever would have bought these for me?"*

Mother was ever the fashion girl, right up to the end!

The Dress

One day Mom and I went shopping. We planned to buy her a new dress for her 89th birthday. We didn't know it then, but it was to be her last birthday. We looked at several dresses but although I thought they were nice, mother didn't like them. Finally, she pointed to a cherry-red suit. She said, *"This is what I want."*

I had my doubts about that specific dress but at Mom's insistence we had her try it on. Perfect!

Sadly in a little more than three months, my mother was buried wearing that beautiful red suit. She was a classy lady right to the very last.

12. SLEEPING

The Effect of Pre-Disease Habits

One of the difficult areas for both the person suffering serious memory loss and the caregiver is in the area of sleep. Sometimes Mom's pre-disease habits impacted her present behaviour. Although mother was often extremely tired, she did not stay asleep long. What was her lifetime habit when she woke up? Usually, she got dressed and then she ate her breakfast. That's what mother still liked to do—get dressed immediately and then eat something.

November 23, 1997: I don't know if I've mentioned before as to the reason why she takes off her nighty. It is because whenever she wakes up at night, she must get dressed for the day. So she takes off her nighty and puts on her housecoat. Then if she falls asleep and awakens again, she frequently puts her nighty over her house-coat. Quite a struggle as her housecoat is bulky. She then is dressed for the day. Interesting—that getting dressed is well coded in her brain.

In the later stages of the disease every time she woke

up, for her it was a new day—whether it was only a fifteen-minute nap, or a longer sleep. After putting on something to wear, the first thing I did when she woke up was to offer her something to eat, or a cup of tea—depending on her need for nourishment. This always had a settling effect.

Desperation

It was two days before Mom's last Christmas. My son Jim, his wife Ginny, and their children were visiting for the holidays. Both Mom and I were extremely tired. At 5:30 p.m. I got her ready for bed, and for a while we both rested. Very soon she was up again, but not for long—she was soon back in bed. I lay down to sleep while Ginny and Jim looked after Mother. At 6:30 p.m. Jim called me. Ginny was in with Mom, but Mother desperately wanted me. I went to her room. She was talking about killing herself: *"There is nothing for me."* I hugged and kissed her, and suggested that she have a cup of tea with me. We went to the kitchen and had our tea. She wanted her mother (usually me!) and said she didn't know where her mother was. I told her perhaps she was resting: *"Everyone has to rest."*

Very occasionally her responses were more placid and resigned, but still sad. One night I asked her if she was tired and wanted to go to bed. *"Yes,"* she said, *"If I'm in bed I'll know where I am."*

When Nothing Works

Sometimes nothing seemed to soothe Mother. Here are excerpts from my journal of such times:

September 22, 1997: I got up between one and two a.m. Went down to Mom. She was sitting on her bed. She said, "I want you to help me. I can't make head or tail out of this" (indicating her Bible). I said, "The reason is you are very tired. Let me put it away and help you back to bed." She allowed me to take the Bible. She pulled at the fringes of her bed covers thinking they were strange. Finally got her lying down but she was distraught—holding herself very tense and not closing her eyes. Gently I held her hands and stroked her face reiterating that she was very tired. "There's lots of night left to sleep" and "There's lots of sleep time." (I never said, "Don't get up," or similar, she only heard the last "Get up.") I could tell I was soothing her but she was far from sleep. So I lay beside her—letting her hold my hand. We lay that way for quite a long time—she was tense—I never did hear her breath relax. I lay with her until about twenty minutes to three and asked her if I could go to my own bed where I could sleep better. She agreed. (Earlier when I asked her the same question she said, "No, you stay here".)

January 1, 1998: Mom up at 2 a.m. I tried every conceivable way to put her back to bed—soothing words—*warm bag—finally crackers and warm water— sitting in a recliner in her bedroom to keep her company. It seemed her mind was programmed to get up and nothing less than getting up would do. Finally, I went back to bed and left her. I tucked her in before I left, but within five minutes I heard her again.

*Note: The warm bag was a therapeutic commercial hot bag that was filled with beans or some similar natural ingredients. When warmed in the microwave oven it stays warm for a long time. I only warmed it for about a minute, so it was nicely warm, but not hot. I then tucked it in by her cheek. This had a very calming effect. I will call it a 'warm bag' in my writing. A 'warm bag' like the one I used for Mom can be purchased in most pharmacies.

January 20, 1998: Mom's restlessness started about 2:30 a.m. I came down at 2:45 and covered her. I thought she would settle but in about twenty minutes it started all over again. I listened for a few minutes then when her pacing slowed, I came downstairs and covered her again. Once more she settled for fifteen to twenty minutes and then she started pacing again. I realized she was not going to settle so I tried to get to sleep myself. Martin covered her (after settling her) at 5 a.m. She went to bed peacefully last night and in a good mood. I have no idea where her sleeplessness comes from or how to prevent it other than medications. She takes one-half an Oxazapam nightly—that works well for first part of the night except when she is extremely agitated. I am afraid that too much medication might produce instability in her walking (sometimes she is unsteady especially when tired.)

She is constantly tired from all the lack of sleep and says such things as this: *"I'm just so tired. I hope I don't wake up."* She was always so sweet, but life was such a burden to her at times.

Efforts to Keep Her Up Later

The thought occurred to me that if she could stay up later in the evening, perhaps she would sleep longer at night, but efforts to keep her up later definitely did not work. If she was tired, it was absolutely essential to get her ready for bed. To illustrate this, here is one of my journal entries:

January 6, 1997: The other night I tried to keep her up a bit longer and she just started coughing and semi-vomiting.

Tiredness also produced tendencies to further confusion and aggression. It was easier to cope with my mother's restlessness at night, although the result was that I was continually tired.

13. SAFETY

Alarms

When Mother lived in the house across the road from both Tony and Robin, and Martin and me, Tony installed an alarm system. Mom had a necklace with an alarm button on it. When she pushed the button, the alarm sounded loudly enough for either household to hear and come to her rescue.

Later when she lived in the seniors' complex, there was also a community alarm system especially designed for elderly people who were living alone. Fortunately there was little need for the alarm systems, but they are certainly worthwhile precautions for early stage dementia when the person is living alone.

Precautions in our Home

When Mother first came to live with us, four years before her death, we were able to leave her for a couple of hours alone. I would leave notes for her: "Donna will come at eleven and get your lunch. Gerry will be home at five and get supper." (Or I might write some other simple instructions or notes so that she was informed.) Of course, because Martin was farming at home, he was continually in and out of the house.

As time progressed, more and more care was needed. The notes now were communications more with her caregivers than with her: "Verta was not feeling well today." "Verta had a good day and enjoyed having tea at the café." As well as other information, these notes would convey safety and health comments.

At night we hooked the basement door high enough so that she could not unlock it and fall down the stairs. Doors leading outside were dead-bolted, and she was physically and mentally unable to unlock them. We turned off the breaker to the stove. We took up all rugs that could trip her. She was accompanied outside as she walked about. We had both a baby monitor and video monitor so that we could check on her well-being during nights.

Tony put up grab bars so she could be as independent and safe as possible. There was a floor-to-ceiling bar beside her bed; two grab bars in the washroom, and two on our back porch.

An occupational therapist came to our home to give us some guidelines to assist her in daily routines and safety measures.

We did everything within our powers to keep her safe. It wasn't enough at the last. She got up from her chair quickly and picked up a TV tray. Martin said, "Here, Grandma let me help you." "No," she said emphatically, *"I will do it myself."* With that she whirled too quickly, lost her balance, and fell and broke her hip.

My Decision

Some decisions are slow in forming; others are instantaneous. One evening, about two years before her death, we went to see a friend who was terminally ill. It was a sad night, and one in which we mentally said goodbye to him. At the same time, I had a nagging feeling that we should not have left Mom home alone. She was in bed—safe we believed—and yet something felt wrong. As I thought through the situation, I realized that we would never leave a two-year-old child alone when he was sleeping nor should we leave my mother who was functioning somewhere near a two year old level. We never did it again. She was always monitored from that time onward. Mother was slowly progressing toward a more dependent state.

14. PERSONAL CARE

Continence & Related Hygiene

I find this area difficult to write about. There are problems associated with Alzheimer's disease that are very personal and private.

Perhaps a few excerpts from our communications records will give an indication of the types of problems that we experienced:

When V. (indicating Verta; my mother) needs to go to the washroom, point to it. You can't say, "Sit on the toilet." You must say, "Take 2 more steps over...now you can sit down," then guide with hand on arm, back or shoulder.

"Doesn't seem to know what to do with toilet tissue after use."

"Bath went well. V. needs close supervision—what used to do doesn't necessarily anymore.

V. needs prompting—each leg of nylon stocking. Keeps leaning off balance.

Mother never really experienced urinary incontinence although I understand that is fairly common with this disease. She did, however, experience occasional periods when her diarrhea was out of control. I remember one time I went in to her. She was in a total mess, with feces all over her body and running down her legs. She was bewildered and angry, *"Who would do this to me? That is a terrible thing to do to someone."* I just quietly washed and cleaned her—diverting her attention as much as possible from this terrible thing that had happened to her.

On occasion, she would sit on the rim of the tub, and use it for a toilet. At other times soiled toilet tissue was found in odd places where she had stashed them. She had trouble comprehending what toilet tissue was to be used for, and often would wipe her nose with it when handed a piece to wipe herself. She needed constant supervision and problems arose if her caregiver did not accompany her at all times. We gave her total care as much as possible, but sometimes other tasks simply had to be done.

Although urinary incontinence was not a problem to my mother, before every outing and periodically throughout the day we encouraged her to use the washroom. At times she was confused at the urination process. The following will illustrate:

October 19, 1997: Before bed she sat on the commode. Didn't urinate. Said, "What is holding it up?" (She referred to her inability to urinate.) *I said, "I don't know." She indicated Granny Pouncy's picture: "I don't think it was that." Then she looked to the left at the light. "It might be that." I said, "Are you finished?" That distracted her.*

Baths

At first when mother lived with us we arranged for weekly baths. As needs changed they became biweekly and then daily. The government Home Care workers gave her the bath and oversaw her dressing. Usually, the baths went well. They had an established routine: "Verta, let's get ready for the day." Then they would lead her to the bathroom where the water had already been prepared. They often would lean down and touch the water temptingly, "Look, here is some nice warm water for your bath." With that they would gently help her off with her housecoat and nightgown and help her into the tub. It seemed to work best if they ignored any negativity mother displayed and just carried on with bathing preparations. Bars and rails had been installed to aid her in getting in and out of the tub with little help.

In the last year of her life, Mom did resist having her bath a few times. One day one of the workers said to her, "I hope you don't give me any tricks today." Mother laughed and replied, *"Tricks?"* Her humour did not always surface though, and I cringed when I heard one of them say, "I'm going to dunk you." Mother always retained a little of her regal bearing and we never used such language with her. How the caregivers approached giving her a bath made a tremendous difference in her resistance or lack of it.

One day she adamantly refused her bath. She came out of the washroom white with anger and very agitated, *"I don't know what is going on, but I will have none of it!"* I guess she must have thought that she was about to be abused, which I'm sure from the distress of the caregiver was not the case. Once more I did not argue with her perceptions. We took her to the bedroom and later on when she had forgotten the incident I gave her a bath.

Dressing and Undressing

I discuss dressing at various times during this book. She went slowly but definitely from being very independent to being very dependent. The following are some journal entries:

September 30, 1996: Verta very vague today. Had bra on over top of slip, undies on sideways, leaving 'tight' red mark on waist and across left thigh. Must have been very uncomfortable. Also difficult to take down.

February 15, 1997: Increasing confusion and paranoia. Last night tried to undress in living room.

15. HEALTH

Because of her age, mother had a number of issues with her health in addition to the dementia: heart failure, vitamin B12 deficiency, Raynaud's disease, diverticulosis, and Meniere's disease. An operation during which a large segment of her stomach was removed happened many years before, and no doubt contributed to diarrhea and malabsorption problems.

Mom had several bouts of pneumonia. I learned that pneumonia does not always present itself the same way in the elderly as in the young. At the onset, she often appeared more confused, disoriented, and much weaker than usual. I recall coming home from work one day. The worker was assisting Mother with each step. I wondered why she believed that Mom needed that much assistance. Then I realized that mother was very ill, and it wasn't long afterwards that we called an ambulance and she was admitted to hospital.

One problem was the need to convey to the hospital staff the importance of the little pill (Serc) to treat the Meniere's disease. The doctor had prescribed it because it seemed to prevent the onset of an incident of the illness. Meniere's is a disease of the inner ear that causes extreme dizziness and vomiting. I told the nurses about the medication and its necessity but somehow it was never given to her. She developed a bout of Meniere's in addition to the pneumonia—problems piled on problems.

The first time she went to hospital the nurses said they would keep her near them so they could monitor her. They called us in distress just after midnight: "Someone will have to sit with your mom twenty-four hours a day or we will have to restrain and medicate her." From then on whenever she was hospitalized, we arranged to stay with her at all times. We had seen my father medicated and restrained and did not want that to happen to mother also.

I relied heavily upon the doctor and pharmacist to help me care for my mother properly. Only once did I fall for some advice from a well-meaning friend. Because of Mom's restlessness at night, someone gave me a Melatonin pill and suggested I give it to her. She slept all right—all night and well into the next afternoon. I worried that I might have inadvertently killed her. I never gave her non-prescription medication again. All medications were prescribed.

Although the memory loss was persistent in its progress, once in a while Mother surprised us. The positive change was probably related to her improved physical health. Note from journal: *Some days she is incredibly better. Much improved. I can hardly believe it.* Unfortunately, such short-lived periods of time were very rare.

16. RESPONDING TO CHANGE

Change is the Only Constant

I have been listening to a motivational tape. It verifies what I found to be true while caring for my mother in her declining years. We need to respond to change because change is the only constant in life.

I studied all the books I could find on Alzheimer's disease, and they were helpful. I put pictures of her grandchildren and great-grandchildren on her bedroom door. As time went by, I wondered how meaningful they were to her. I asked her "Would you rather have pictures of the children or of flowers?" She said, *"Flowers."* Of course, the actual children were important to Mom but the pictures had ceased to have any meaning.

I put up a bulletin board close to her bedroom. At first she enjoyed the pictures and information I posted on it, but soon she lost interest. In fact, she started taking things off and putting them in her Bible. I had to discover a new way to keep her in touch with her family and her own history.

October 5, 1997: Comparing Mom to a year ago—last

year we took her to Kamloops (about 90 miles away)... lunch at Fran and Lorne's (grandchildren's home). Shopping at Mall, bought winter coat and boots. Now an hour or two ride in a car completely plays her out. It's good to have milestones to compare to, as it's hard to track on a day-to-day basis. She is so precious—I hate to see this downward trend.

Emotional Response

Usually mother's overwhelming emotion to her disease was distress.

November 2, 1997: (Mom) woke up again about 8 p.m. "Why am I so stupid? Why can't I remember anything? Why can't I remember anybody?" Me: "Do you remember me?" Mom: "A little. Kind of, but I—don't remember anything." Me: "Do you remember the babies?" Answer: "I like the babies but I can't really remember them." Mom motioning to glass of water and saucer: "I can't remember them. Finally she said, "Gordie." I said, "Yes, Gordie was here. You remember Gordie?" She motioned around. "But I don't remember anything. I don't like to be like this." I said, "I know you don't. It's frustrating. You are getting old; you've been sick, and you're really tired. You'll feel a lot better in the morning." Got her off to bed—'warm bag'—tender words, etc. Hope she sleeps now.

November 29, 1997: Her mix-up is a little incredible at times. Last night she kept pointing to the trees on her TV tray and asking who they belonged to. She was upset because she said her man asked her for money. I explained he had died almost 10 years ago and maybe she had dreamed it. She kept going over it. You can't get her out of an idea except by redirection. It also helped that it was time to give her Oxazepam pill.

December 19, 1997: Now I'm trying to calm her: "Nothing to do. I don't know anything. I'm stupid. I look around and I don't see anything I can do. Do you look after me? Why don't I know anything? What sickness have I had? I wish I knew what I was doing, but I haven't a clue." Sad and nothing I can do to fix.

Part of the stress that I experienced was in recognizing her distress, and trying to constantly minimize it by gentle words and actions and by redirection. Mom's distress was very real and vicious. I called her illness the 'Vicious Disease'.

A Book of Memories

Mother was in a depressed mood. *"I am no good. I have never done anything good in my life. I am no good to anyone."*

I was grateful that at least Mom was able to verbalize her feelings—many people with severe memory loss are unable to do so. Now I had a dilemma. How could I help Mom recognize what a remarkable woman she was and all the exceptional things she had achieved?

Mother had always been an outstanding woman. Someone told me when I was an adolescent that if I grew up to be half the woman my mother was, I would be a great woman.

Mother was a firm believer in "Try another way"—if one way doesn't work then make it work with a different approach. As children we were taught, "Whatever you do, do with your might. Things done by halves are never done right." That was my mother—the most loving and capable person I knew. Yet here she was in the depths of despair because she could not remember any of those wonderful things she had done, and the person she had been.

In order that she might get an idea of what an important and talented person she was, I got a photo album with plastic sheets that lifted so that I could insert whatever I desired. I printed and used simple language as if I were doing it for a child in grade two. On pages of a pretty writing pad I printed out the simple story of her life. I told of her accomplishments, her parents, her marriage, her children, and anything I thought would provide happy memories for her.

I can see her yet, poring over her book every day, reading each page, and giving a little laugh, *"Somebody thought I was good."* This book soothed her more than anything else and is certainly a strategy worth noting. I could not have given my mother a more precious gift— the gift of self-esteem and perhaps even a little memory. If I could live those years over again, I would not give up that opportunity to give something of value to my precious mother.

Flexibility First

Well, maybe flexibility isn't first. I think that love and gentleness are first, but flexibility is very important. Even her personal book that meant so much to her had to be changed periodically. If something I had written bothered her, I simply removed it. Fortunately I had chosen to put the information in a photo album with overlying plastic pages. That enabled me to easily remove or add some new information.

There are many illustrations of flexibility described throughout this book. I don't believe there was one area of her life in which adaptations did not have to be made frequently. Those adaptations signify the necessity for caregivers to be extremely flexible. The food that she was willing to eat varied and I had to adapt to her changing desires. Her ability to dress herself frequently changed too. The activities that greatly enhanced her life were in a constant state of flux. For some of us who tend to be very organized these types of changes can be a serious problem. When we are extremely organized we like to control our lives, and sometimes the lives of those around us. Certainly, personality tests reveal that flexibility is a characteristic that we all naturally have to different degrees. I tend to see flexibility and organization as opposite sides of the coin. If you are extremely organized then you will naturally be less flexible, and vice versa. I also believe that it is possible to strengthen weak areas in our personalities. I hope that I will prove the necessity to develop strong flexibility skills, as these skills are greatly valuable to the person you are serving. It will also make your job much easier!

Although there was a gradual decline in memory and functioning ability, there were variations. Possibly it was related to her health or fatigue. A factor that impacted her functioning was her levels of vitamin B12. She had a deficiency in it, and after her monthly shot she improved slightly. Another difference showed up when the doctor gave her a prescription for antibiotics. After a course of them she seemed much more alert for a few days. I am sorry that I did not arrange a full assessment of her health and mental capabilities early in the course of the disease. Because of my experience in human services I knew better, but I was always afraid of offending my mother. If I were able to go back in time and change one thing about mother's care, I would arrange for her to receive a thorough medical and geriatric assessment. Certainly she went to the doctor for help frequently, but an assessment in a geriatric facility was available and we did not take advantage of it.

Perhaps the main factor in her functioning ability was the love, gentleness, and respect everyone gave her. It was easy for me to see how aggression and agitation might develop if we did not give her what her soul needed most. How easily we forget the maxim, "Do unto others, as you would have them do unto you." Yet, it is vitally important.

Just Plain Sad

One night I heard her in the middle of the night. I checked the video monitor in our bedroom and knew mother needed me.

I entered her room and with great bewilderment she said, *"Where am I? Where am I?"* I tried to explain and then said, "Mom, isn't there anything you recognize?" *"Nothing,"* she said.

We had filled her room with as many valued, personal possessions we could. I said, "Look, Mom, here are all your treasures." As I pointed them out, Mom looked around with puzzlement, and with disdain she replied simply, *"Treasures?"* I knew then that her treasures meant nothing to her. The change had come gradually but it had come, and the only thing to do was to accept it and move on.

A Familiar Face

Can you imagine what it must feel like to wake up in a strange room every morning and not recognize anything or remember how you got there, or even why you are there? What if you met hundreds of people and didn't recognize anyone. How would you feel? Then can you visualize how you would feel in these strange surroundings amongst all these strange people, and you see one person that you recognize? Oh, you don't know the name, but somehow there is something about that person—you know you have found a friend.

Sometimes when Mom and her companion and I were at the same gathering, Mom would catch a glimpse of me across a crowded room and her face would light up in a beautiful smile. Even though she didn't know my name or who I was, that smile spoke volumes.

17. RELATIONSHIPS

Are you my Brother?

Mother was agitated. No, mother was extremely angry. She said to me, *"You know what your husband said to me? He said that my brother was my son. Why is he saying that to me? A mother could never forget her son—he is my brother!"* Mom was referring to her only son, Frank.

I suppose the confusion came because she had mothered many of her brothers and sisters when she was only a child herself, or perhaps her memory became stuck prior to her giving birth. Her earlier memories were the most dominant. But for Frank it was very hurtful and dramatic.

I tried to calm Mom. "Mom", I gently said, "He *is* your son. I remember when he was born. I remember when you had him. You can trust me."

Mom said nothing. That night as I helped her get ready for bed she said very angrily, *"Do you know what your husband said to me? He said my brother is my son. Why would he do such a terrible thing?"*

'OK', I thought to myself, 'so this is truly what mother believes. No one is going to change her mind. We will go with her perceptions. We will not argue with her. It is useless.'

My Identity

Mother's confusion as to her relation to family members did not stop with my brother. One night Mom and I were sitting in the living room. She was increasingly becoming agitated and I didn't know why. Finally she said, *"Where is Mother?"* I replied, "Oh, darling, your mother died. She is not living." Greatly alarmed Mom said, *"But she was just here. I saw her."* At the moment I didn't understand why that would seem true to her, but I soon realized that I was slipping in and out of being 'mother' to my mother.

One night Mother did not want to go to bed. She told me she was waiting for her mother. Mom was clearly very distressed and worried. I said to her, "Oh, your mother has gone out for the evening. She will be here when you wake up in the morning." Mother happily went to bed and I, her pseudo-mother, was truly with her when she woke up in the morning.

It was really strange how when most of the time she perceived me as her mother, occasionally a little sliver of memory would break through the haze. How good it was, but it lasted momentarily and was extremely rare. I had to keep in my mind that whoever I was, she loved and appreciated me.

November 11, 1997: Mom went in the big chair—all wrapped up—slept. Woke up—came out to kitchen. I asked her if she'd like coffee: "Yes"—If she'd like toast: "Yes". Got both for her. Suddenly she animatedly said, "You're Gerry!" It's good to be recognized by your mother. She knows I'm someone who cares. One time she said to me, "When Gerry comes she'll know what to do."

February 15, 1998: In her stress she seemed to be more aware. Some things almost seem clearer—like she was calling me "Gerry". At the lunch table a visitor said that there weren't many Gerrys around (to take care of family elders). Mom said, "And I keep Gerry in line!"

One day Mom said to me: "*Where is Gerry?*" I hesitated a moment and then said, "Who am I?" Mom said quizzically, "*Gerry?*" A minute later she said again, "*Where is Gerry?*" Sometimes Mother asked if I was the one over her. I guess she recognized me as the one responsible for her care.

Occasionally Mom would mix her identity up with mine. When she was ill, I went in to her. She said, "*Gerry is sick. Is Gerry going to be all right?*"

January 6, 1997: Last night Mom was looking at a picture of Joyce, Faith (Alica), and myself (my sisters and I). I asked her who looked like her. She pointed at me in the middle, "Her—my mother. I look like my mother" (even though my name 'Gerry' was on the picture). I guess I am firmly placed as her mother.

January 30, 1997: Mother showed me her picture again in the photo album. I said, "Isn't that nice. Who is it?" She said, "You" (indicating me). Then she said, "Maybe it's my mother. It looks a bit like my mother."

November 23, 1997: I asked Mom if she'd like to do something. She said, "No, I am just sitting here waiting for her. She may come or she may not." No one is here beside Mom, Martin, and me. She keeps looking for her mother. (Me at a different time!)

January 26, 1997: Mom gave me the photo book with her picture and said, "Here, this is yours. This is your picture." (It is a picture of her.)

This mix-up in our identities remained to the very last. *February 27, 1998, when in hospital during Mom's final illness she said to me: "I am dying" interspersed with "Gerry is dying." Yesterday she patted my hand and said, "Are you OK? Are you muddled up?" This mix-up of her identity with mine reminds me about a time a few months ago when she was vomiting. I left her and came back to check. She said, "How is Gerry? I think she was sick."*

Mom's Father

Mother's dad was a very big man—huge in fact. Time has erased exactly how tall he was but we know he was a giant of a man, both tall and broad. My mother adored her father. He had an Irish brogue and was very deaf. Mother often told how she was daddy's little girl. She went around with him, interpreting his speech to others, and relaying their message to him.

He died when Mother was in her twenties. On New Year's Day the family were invited out for dinner. Grandpa said, "Go without me. I am not feeling very well." When they returned they found that he had died. My mother was devastated and never fully recovered. As children we were not allowed to celebrate New Year's Day because that was the day our grandfather died.

In my childhood our family had only one picture of my grandfather. He was standing eye to eye with some draft horses. In Mom's declining years an aunt sent me a different picture. It was larger than the first. Mother took the picture and put it close to her heart. *"I am never going to let him go," she insisted. She would only barely let it out of her sight when she went to bed. It was then that I realized that the picture became in reality her father. I quietly put it away and she forgot.*

Martin, My Husband

(The following is a little story I wrote some years ago about Mother and Martin:)

Verta watched the young man. He had curly brown hair, and startling blue eyes. His step was quick and lively, his manner gentle and kind. Verta noticed that he always seemed to be working. What a wonderful person, she thought, and what a good choice for her unmarried daughter. Wisely she said nothing as she watched the budding romance.

Verta was my mom, and she was ill in the hospital when Martin and I walked in together.

"Guess what, Mom," I said.

"I know," she said, *"you and Martin are engaged. I picked him out for you long ago."*

So she became the beloved mother-in-law to that very special young man.

Years passed and Verta made sure that her son-in-law

had the best—pies, biscuits, and delicious homemade raisin buns.

Still more years passed, and Verta was now in her eighties. Martin was no longer young. His curly hair was now white and much scarcer. He worked as hard as ever, but his steps were accompanied with daily pain caused by a near-fatal accident when he was just 34 years old. Just the same, he was still that special, gentle, hard-working person.

Verta, though, was gradually losing ground. She was still gentle and loving but her memory and health were beginning to fail, and she came to live with us on the farm.

Day after day he tenderly shared in her care, even though she no longer recognized him. That didn't matter to him; he just kept on loving her.

One day she watched at the kitchen window as he raked the fallen leaves under the big, old maple tree. Up and down he jumped on his old pick-up truck, as he packed the leaves he had just thrown on it. Verta stared in fascination and utter amazement.

"Up and down. Up and down he goes, and him crippled and all," Verta voiced her admiration.

Verta may have recognized him a bit when he wore his suit and tie, but those farming coveralls, and that tattered hat were something else again.

One day he was walking around the yard dressed in his usual farming garb when Verta saw him out of her bedroom window.

"Look," she said with consternation, *"there is that man again. Shall we let him in?"*

"Oh, darling, that man is my husband. I am married to him," I said, as gently as I could.

Verta looked at me with poorly concealed amusement, as she half covered her mouth.

"Oh, you poor dear. I'm sorry. I shouldn't laugh but I can't help it. I'm so sorry."

Although Verta has now been gone for several years, I can still see her clearly, and that gentle hard-working man is still my husband. They will live in my heart forever.

Martin's help was absolutely essential to my ability to adequately care for Mother. He supported me in many ways, caring for her at times, and in other ways encouraging me. He was very kind to her, although she did not always treat him with the dignity and respect he deserved. When she said, "Thank you" to him this was important and special.

Husband Harry (My Dad)

Sometimes Mom vehemently denied ever being married to a man named Harry, and other times she looked for him. He had died several years previously and she had dealt with her grief at the time.

Sometimes she would look at Dad's picture and call him Frank (her son). Somehow she knew family names but had a difficult time connecting names to people or pictures of people.

Dad had a picture taken when he was in the Royal Canadian Air Force in the Second World War. One day Mother pointed to that picture, in which Dad looked very stern and unsmiling. She said, *"That bothers me. I don't like it."* She insisted that I take it down.

Her special book that I made for her told about her marriage to Dad and all about her four children, and the family's life together. Each time Mom read it she seemed surprised. I had pictures around of Dad and of the two of them together. One time she commented on what nice people they were, although she did not seem to recognize who they were. Yet somewhere in the deep recesses of her mind there seemed a little spark of memory that popped up once in a long while.

Amanda and Alyssa

My 17-year-old granddaughter, Amanda, came for a visit. Mother seemed very aware that Amanda was somehow special, yet she was very disturbed. She thought, because of Amanda's small stature, that she was a child. She repeatedly asked, *"Where is your mother?"* I explained that Amanda was seventeen and that she (my mother) was married at seventeen. Mother's agitation quickly changed emphasis. She became concerned that perhaps Amanda would go through life without a man to love her. Mother quickly retorted, *"Have you a beau?"* When Amanda indicated "No", mother said with great animation, *"Well, you better get with it then!"*

Mom thought Amanda was just wonderful and instructed me to give her anything she wanted, and to look after her. After telling me what to do for Amanda, she looked at me, *"You be sure you look after yourself. You have everything you want."* Mom was able to give and receive love and that was very special.

Another of her great-granddaughters, Alyssa, was just approaching her teen years when Mother was at the height of her illness. Our son Jim, his wife Ginny and their family were visiting us. Mother must have been observing Alyssa very closely and one morning she went on a talking jag. She told me how much Alyssa loved babies. She also told me how her mother had eight babies and how Alyssa had helped right along with her, looking after the babies. Of course, this was impossible. Mom's parents, and most of their children, had long since died and Alyssa was just a child. Just the same,

Mom's observations about Alyssa were accurate—she loved and gave great care to little ones.

All the Family

Despite all her dementia, paranoia, and confusion Mother still seemed to epitomize love. One day she looked at a picture of our whole family and said, *"I want you to get them all here. I want to see them. Get Dad too."* This love extended to all her children, and descendants, and beyond. If she heard her maiden name, 'Huston', she would perk up and listen intently. Somehow she knew that whoever owned that name was special to her.

Our Sons

Mother had a loving relationship with our children and their wives. This was no doubt because she lived close to us and finally in our home, and our family did a great deal to help her. Our son Jim had been very close in earlier years but now lived farther away so she was not quite as familiar with him.

Tony helped her with many things, including doing much of her business for her. He would often pop into our place for lunch, so she knew him as well as she knew anyone, and loved him.

Gordie and his wife Karen often came to visit and brought their two small children—she called them the "little ones". They were very important to her. She admired Gordie greatly. One day after he had been visiting us, she said of him (although she called him by the wrong names): *"Andy is very good. He's so good to the children."* Later on she said of him again: *"Tom is so good. He is good with the children."* (Mother always had a great appreciation for anyone who treated children gently and with loving care.)

January 19, 1998: I just got off the phone with Gordie, and I told Mom who I had been talking to. She said, *"Oh, I like Gordie. He's a nice person. He does the right things...He's always been so good. He is so gentle and so nice to everyone."* I must tell Gordie. We all need the love and approval of the 'matriarch' of the family.

18. PERCEPTIONS

Perceptions and Alzheimer's Disease

It is my opinion that perceptions play a major role in the confusion, paranoia, and even aggression of persons with Alzheimer's disease. For instance, when my mother was extremely agitated over her perceived missing jewelry, she firmly believed that it had been stolen. Her ability to reason had been destroyed, and she remained firm in her perception.

When she perceived that her son was her brother or that I was her mother, nothing that anyone said made any difference. Her perceptions were fixed.

She believed pictures and TV images were actual people, and she would accept no other answer. Her reality was her reality, and those perceptions could not be altered by anyone.

November 11, 1997: Mother was looking at pictures of children in a book. One of them had very little clothes on. Mom said, "Here, I'll give this to you (the book). I haven't anything to put on her."

The images on television also became very real. One of her caregivers often put on a home video, thinking it would amuse her to see the grandchildren. One day I came in and mother seemed tired. "Mom, would you like me to turn off the TV?" *"No,"* she replied, *"Let the children play; they are having so much fun."*

The following is an excerpt from my journal that will illustrate how disturbing pictures could be:

August 8, 1997: Mom very tired and very confused.

Last night I brought out a picture of Dad and her. I thought she would want to see it so I sat it on the table in front of her supper. She wouldn't eat any of her supper. When I talked to her about not eating she said, "He (indicating Dad) is watching me." I said, "Would you like me to take the picture away?" She replied, "No, I don't know who would want it." I responded, "But if it's bothering you maybe it would be better to take it away." Mom: "No, he wants to come out." Me: "He can't come out, he's dead." Mom: "Dead", she said in alarm. I said, "Why don't I just move it into the other room?" She said okay but still didn't eat her supper.

I had furnished my mother's bedroom with as many of her possessions that I could reasonably get in it. On one wall was a picture of her grandmother and grandfather. *"Take them down"*, Mom said, *"She is too cranky."* As I obeyed I motioned to another picture—a large portrait of Mom's mother-in-law that hung above her bed and asked her if she would like me to take it down too. *"No,"* Mom replied, *"She just smiles at me all night long. She is so nice. She looks after me."* So Grandma's picture remained.

Self Perception

Mother seemed to have very little perception of herself—her body, and her capabilities. She often referred to herself in the second person and might not refer to herself in the right gender: *"She wants--,"* or *"He doesn't know what to do."*

Before she was diagnosed and before we realized how much her memory and understanding had deteriorated, she made some statements that amused us at the time. She was living in a seniors' apartment complex. The fire department had talked to the seniors about fire safety. With all seriousness, mother said, *"I'm not worried. I'll just have Tony hang a rope from my balcony and I'll shinny down it."* We all laughed at the mental picture of my eighty-five-year old, fragile mother shinnying down from the second floor balcony. She indignantly responded, *"Of course, I can shinny. I have always been able to shinny."* Whether or not this story illustrates impaired perception or if it just shows how resilient and inventive Mother was, I still don't know. Fortunately, she never had to prove her 'shinnying' ability.

One day, Mom asked how old she was. When I told her she was eighty-nine, she was amazed, and said, *"Oh dear."* In childlike innocence she sometimes asked me, *"Am I good?"*

Reflections

There is a condition in Alzheimer's disease called sundowning. About the time of sundown each day, the patient becomes increasingly confused and disoriented. Although I had heard of the condition before, I had never felt its full impact. Every night as evening approached I noticed that mother became more agitated. But why? My curiosity was whetted. My previous experience working with both seniors and with persons who had mental disabilities made me want to delve into this mystery. Perhaps she was tired or maybe the day's frustrations had become too much of a burden.

I gradually became aware that there was one specific thing that greatly agitated Mom. It was the reflections in the windows and that came off the TV. When an individual walked across the room, his reflection seemed to walk through the window and cross the room towards you. I solved that problem by drawing the curtains and drapes as soon as reflections appeared each evening. However, all problems with reflections could not be solved that easily: TV screens, stove oven windows, and a myriad of other little objects reflected lights and shadows. Mother tended to escape by retiring early, stating that she's going to bed so she'll know where she is. Of course, going to bed didn't necessarily stop the confusion.

I Never Had a Bite

Mother continually wanted to go somewhere and do something. With a restless energy she liked to fill her life with excitement. We hired someone to take her out each day. At first she went to various community activities. Finally they became too confusing. So usually she and her caregiver went out for lunch or for tea.

One day when she came home from eating lunch in a café, I asked her if she had enjoyed it. She replied that everyone was eating all around her, but she never had a bite. No one would give her anything. Of course I knew this was only her perceptions and not reality. "Mom, would you like a bite to eat now?" I asked. *"Oh, yes."* This happened frequently but she was always relieved and grateful no matter what I gave her—perhaps only a cup of tea, a quarter of a banana, or a couple of crackers. Again it was a matter of respecting her and her perceptions and refusing to argue. Her memory was simply her memory, and I recognized that I could not change reality as she saw it.

Ownership

Mother had almost no conception of true ownership. She believed that everything belonged to her or to her mother. If she had been placed in a facility it was plain to all of us who were with her daily, that she would have had a great deal of trouble. No doubt that she would have been restrained either physically or chemically (or both). This, I did not want. I had seen it before with my dad. I did put her name on a waiting list to a facility in case we were forced to institutionalize her, but fortunately we never had to do it.

The following excerpt from my journal will give you an idea of how the situation was:

August 18, 1997: She thinks it is her home. One day she said of my husband: "Who does he think he is? Does he think he owns this or something?" I wanted to say, "Well, he does"—but again I realize that there would be no advantage to setting the record straight. Perhaps the greatest wisdom is to accept the person's perceptions as truth—knowing full well they are not reality. I don't lie per se, but acknowledge the perception. When she is worried about visitors I say: "They are all cared for. Everything's fine."

The Relationship between Actions & Perceptions

Actions are often based on perceptions. I remember once I was in a church meeting. Without warning the church was attacked. I thought, "Someone is shooting at the church." Without considering the risk to myself, I ran outside to confront the attackers. Later I discovered that it was stones that hit the windows of the church, not bullets. We were not in any serious danger. I acted solely on my perceptions. My perceptions were that we were being shot at, and I acted on my false reality. Some people will flee and hide in the face of danger; other people, like me in that situation, will fight back.

People with Alzheimer's will do the same. Their reality, although often not based on fact, is so strong that they refuse to be dissuaded from their beliefs, and often their response is to fight back—we call it aggression, to them it is just simply survival.

How does a loving caregiver or family member deal with this distressing situation? I found that in most situations I acted on my mother's perceptions. If she declared that she had eaten nothing all day, I gently said, "Would you like a cup of tea and some banana?" Immediately her distress at being starved was gone.

Although I knew she had eaten just one-half hour ago, it was a simple matter to act on her perceptions. Most of the time this was possible, and it was done in a way that did not harm her physically and helped her emotionally.

Occasionally we had to ignore her perceptions for her own welfare. When she was eighty-nine she fell in our living room and broke her hip. The doctor told me that she needed an operation. "She will not survive an operation," I said. "She will not survive if she does not have an operation," he rejoined. So I agreed. She survived the operation but needed an IV. She repeatedly pulled out the needle, so the nurses tied her arm to the bed. Mother was totally distressed. "They are killing me," she angrily repeated many times. In her efforts to survive she turned to me, her perceived mother. *"You're my very own mother and you stand there and let them kill me,"* she accused me. That was very hard but I tried to ignore her distress because I knew her life depended on the IV. I did not, however, argue with her, as experience had taught me that her behaviour would escalate if I argued.

Mother's Apron

Mom gave me an apron that she had made, embroidered, and finished with a crocheted frill. It was lovely. I really treasured that apron and wore it often. Once when I was wearing it, Mom said in her sternest voice, *"Take off that apron. It belongs to Mother."* In those moments she did not seem to recognize me as the mother who helped her every day. At first I tried to reason with her, "Oh, Mother said I could borrow it." Mom would not accept that explanation. After several attempts to get away with wearing it, I finally hid the apron. That was much easier than dealing with the issue.

The same sort of thing happened about my husband's sweater. Close to ten years previously my father had died. Mom gave Martin one of Dad's sweaters. Martin had worn it for several years with no incidents. Then one day Mom indignantly said to him, *"That's my man's sweater. What did you do with him? Why did you take his sweater?"* It was easy to see by her behaviour that she suspected foul play. It became prudent to put the sweater out of her sight.

It seemed that although her memories were somehow blocked, once in a while a little bit would escape. Something would trigger a slight break-through.

People have said to me: "I don't feel sorry for the people who have Alzheimer's because they don't know anything. I feel sorry for their family." I don't agree. Certainly sympathize with the family, but I went every step through the disease with my mom and I recognize the distress that she had daily. It is a great gift to be able to empathize—to mentally get into the other person's skin; feel what they feel, and perceive things as they perceive them.

Difficulties Regarding Size

Our two youngest grandchildren were frequent visitors to our home. They played in the sandbox or rode their bikes. When the oldest, Sarina, was just three and one half years old she had a tiny two-wheeler with training wheels. Sometimes the family would go home and leave the bike at our place, as it was a safe place for her to practice. Several times Mom claimed that the bike was her man's and became very possessive. The truth was that Dad was a motorcyclist—so this small bike had a tiny semblance of reality although it was much, much smaller and far less complex.

As I have said, Mother's father was a huge man— broad in build and very tall. In Mom's mind he grew and grew. One day she told me that her dad was so big that he had to get down on his hands and knees and crawl to get through a door—slivers of reality and a great many misperceptions. We never argued with her perceptions, always treating her with respect and dignity.

Several years before mother's dementia became acute, she lived near us. Tony and Robin lived across the road, and our house was a short distance to the north. At that time, Robin had a little dog named Binkie. While Robin was at work, Binkie often spent time with Mom. During the day the dog would trot across the road to Mother's house, and sleep in a specially covered chair. When Robin and Tony's son, Steven, came home from school the dog would leave the house and go to the road to meet the school bus. Through all that time Mother and Binkie developed a very special relationship.

One day Binkie gave birth to a litter of puppies. For some reason I have long ago forgotten, the basket of puppies was left at our house—but Binkie was outside. The dog was very agitated and repeatedly went to Mom. In and out the house she went. Finally, mother realized that Binkie was trying to give her a message. Dancing back and forth, Binkie led Mom to our house where the mystery was solved. Mom helped Binkie save the day, and so the bond between them grew.

A few years later, when Mother's disease was well pronounced, Binkie wandered away and became lost. Martin and I went out hunting for her while Mother remained in the car. As time went by, Mom's stories of Binkie became more and more interesting. Mother told how she had walked and walked calling for her dog, but she never came. In Mom's stories Binkie had grown from a very small size to be gigantic! (Incidentally and sadly, little Binkie was never found.)

Mother had always loved animals of all kinds, as well as birds. She sometimes nursed little birds back to health when they had been injured. At times she even trained an occasional bird to eat out of her hand. Her love of all creatures great and small carried on throughout her dementia—even though she displayed miscomprehensions about their size, shape, and colour. I'm not sure about the usual reaction to pets by persons with Alzheimer's disease. It probably would depend on their previous responses to animals, and whether or not fear had been a factor. It certainly would be worth testing someone's responses because often a pet provides a great deal of comfort. I remember when my father was in an extended care hospital, he loved and received great comfort from a cat that liked to lie on his bed.

Writing about Mom's love of animals and birds reminds me of a little incident that happened recently. I was spending a 'Grandma Day' with my granddaughter, Morgan, who was seven years old at the time. Although she was only a very small child when mother was alive, she treasures each little memory and the stories she hears of Grandma Pouncy. As Morgan and I were talking she said to me, "Grandma Pouncy had a gift. She held birds in her hand." Morgan paused and added: "All my grandmas have gifts." And then Morgan looked very thoughtful and with a look of puzzlement asked, "Grandma, what is your gift?" I did some quick thinking and then replied, "Morgan, my gift is that I love my grandchildren." Relieved, Morgan sighed, "Yes Grandma, your gift is you have us."

Closed Doors

I mentioned elsewhere that we closed her closet door at night so she would not try to dress herself. However, that was not the only door that we closed. The following journal excerpt will explain the situation:

January 23, 1998: Have I mentioned that if a door is closed for Mother, it is as if the room beyond does not exist. We have been closing her closet door for months now with the knowledge that she will not try to open it. She will still open her bedroom door—but if in the night she goes out of her room and closes the door she may not find her way (without help) back into her bedroom. For a couple of months now we have been closing the dining-room and living-room doors at nights—that way she keeps her wanderings to the hall and kitchen.

19. DEALING WITH DEATH

Her Brother

How does a person who has trouble with memory, relationships, and coping with day-to-day living deal with death? The answer is with huge difficulties.

Mother's brother, Keith, had been ill for some time, and we took her to see him in the hospital. Then he died. I felt it was my duty to tell her about his death. I thought she had a right to know, but I knew she would get very confused. What better way to tell you the degree of her confusion than to give you some of the entries from my journal:

September 3, 1997: After Donna left, I told Mom about Keith's death. She was very sad and talked about what a good boy he always was (he was seventy-four). Accurately she said, "We saw him and I knew he was sick." So she had some memories of him. I saw tears in her eyes. Before supper she seemed to have forgotten, but after supper she picked up Keith's picture and the following note:

Keith Huston

Funeral, Friday, 2 p.m.

Verta will go to it.

(When I wrote 'Verta will go to it,' I thought I was just giving her information and because it was written she would remember it better. That proved to be a very poor decision as the continuation of my journal entry of September 3, 1997, describes:)

She said (when I mentioned he was her brother). "He was not my brother. He's my cousin." His name is not Huston; it's something else—the same as Jim's." I responded "Meggait?" She replied, "Yes. He asked for me—no one else. He said he wanted me to come. I will need someone to take me. I want Frank (Mom's son) to take me." (Unfortunately, Frank could not come to the funeral because of his employment, but of course she forgot that she had asked for him.) I was afraid of the consequences of telling her—but felt it was her right to know. She was adamant about going to the funeral.

Later on the same day I made these entries:

Mom said, "He wrote in there, and told me to help him. I didn't get a chance to do anything. It was funny. He wanted me to help him, but there was nothing put out. I want you to go through the papers and see if you can figure. They wanted me to help them. They want people to talk more. In one place he said, 'Verta can come. You'll find it there." Confusion obviously about Keith's death and funeral. Her mind is so very fragile. In retrospect, I should not have written, "Verta will go." I thought I was just giving her information, but she perseverated about it. It's impossible to make the right decision at all times.

September 4, 1997: Mom didn't mention Keith at all, so I thought she had forgotten, but she told her Home Support worker that there were two boys and one of them died. She said she was with him and helped him.

September 5, 1997: Keith's funeral...She seemed pale, confused, and overwhelmed. Very fragile. Then (after the funeral) ...she met the family and enjoyed that.

September 6, 1997: Today Mom remembers something. Just what is hard to determine. Brought Keith's picture to her and she said, "Keith, I never knew it was Keith." (Of course we had told her many times.) "He looks exactly like someone else." She is trying in her own way to cope with her loss.

Dear Mom, it was so difficult for her. When strong emotions came, they seem to be accompanied by little sparks of memory but still she was confused. Sometimes gentle words and loving ways failed to take away all the grief in life, let alone the pain of this vicious disease.

Her Husband

My Dad died in 1988. At first Mom remembered and did the normal grieving, but as time passed she forgot. Yet every once in a while she seemed to vaguely remember 'her man'. Twice one evening almost nine years after he had passed away, she asked for him: *"He was around here and now I can't find him. I saw him and he's gone."* I told her about Dad's death both times. She showed total surprise. It's her only misperception that I tried to correct, as the truth was easier for her to handle than for her to constantly search for him. (Sometimes, she thought he had run off with another woman, neglecting her, or that she was neglecting him.)

20. PARANOIA

I came to believe strongly that from the point of view of the person with severe memory loss, paranoia was perfectly natural and inevitable. Loss of memory involves loss of any knowledge of personal possessions. Sometimes mother believed that everything in the house belonged to her or her mother, therefore, if anyone picked up something (no matter how simple), according to her they were stealing. Her gentle and kind nature probably protected us from even more paranoia, but even Mom had her breaking point.

She understood neither her physical nor her mental problems and constantly thought people were playing cruel tricks on her. *"Who would do this awful thing to me? Why are they so cruel?"* How does a loving caregiver explain such things? Often I couldn't, and only kindness and gentleness had any effect on quieting her. Love and patience helped when nothing else could.

Here are some entries in my journal that may illustrate these points:

September 1, 1997: I'm glad she is some better physically; unfortunately, it does not cure memory loss and resulting confusion, agitation, and paranoia. Yesterday she was accusing someone of stealing her camera. It probably belonged to a visitor and he was just picking up his own camera, but she doesn't accept correction.

September 2, 1997: She told me that the man just took something from in front of her (implication was that he stole it). "I paid for it myself. It was mine." I have no idea what the something was—probably something Martin moved from her TV tray so he could put her breakfast on it. I explained, held her hand, soothed her, gave her the personal book I had prepared for her, and finally settled her.

November 16, 1997: Lots of paranoia. "Someone is taking Mother's things." I tried to reassure her that no one in our family is like that, they are just helping, but she would not accept—very angry and upset with no justification. Somewhere today she misunderstood actions.

8 p.m. Mom off to bed. While having snack said things like men are crawling into bed with her. I explained that there was no one here who would do that. She said, "There is and you know who." She maybe dreamed it because this often occurs after she has slept.

December 26, 1997: Christmas come and gone. Mom had spells of enjoyment and spells of anger. Usually I can figure it out. I had put out general treats for all to enjoy, which they did, but she thought everyone was eating her food. I knew confusion would cause disorientation, anger, and paranoia—which it did. This is a vicious disease.

We all have a choice:
Kick and scream at our lot in life or
Adapt and alleviate the negative situation

PART THREE

THE ESSENCE OF

HER PERSON

1. SPARKS OF HER FORMER SELF

Despite her serious loss of memory, the perceptions that did not correspond to reality, and her lack of comprehension, there always remained a spark of the essence of the mother that I had always known and loved. It was true she did not know my name, but she knew that I was someone who loved her and she always loved me back.

She had always been a lady of class and style, and despite all the problems, both physical and mental, Mother somehow managed to maintain that noble stature. Mother loved to dress well. She loved people and invariably wanted to help them. She always wanted to be active and adventuresome—music and a good time excited her. She loved nature and God. All these things were still a part of her personality when her life ground to a halt.

2. SPIRITUALITY

Mom was a devoted Christian who spent many years loving and studying the Bible. Her Bible was perhaps her most precious possession. Towards the end I realized that she was losing even that—not her faith, but the knowledge of what the Bible was. One day she brought me her Bible. With a great deal of puzzlement, she said, "I've looked and looked and I can't find anything in it." At first I thought she didn't understand the words but as her confusion continued I realized that she had mixed up her Bible and her purse. She was really looking for money.

Until close to the end, she went to church with us and seemed comforted by it. She did have trouble with the concept of Christmas though. It was her last Christmas in 1997. My husband brought in a spruce tree for me to decorate. *"Get that thing out of here"* my mother said disgustedly. *"It doesn't belong here. It belongs outside."*

"Oh, Mom," I replied, "It's Christmas and we are celebrating Jesus' birthday." Her demeanor improved immediately. Excitedly she exclaimed, *"Oh, is he coming to our house?"*

Another time as the Christmas tree sat decorated in the living room, Mom said, *"That looks funny—just sitting there and sitting there."* I responded, *"Isn't it pretty?"* Mom: *"Yes it's pretty, but it does nothing and I don't see anything I can do. I don't know what it's for or why we do it."* Unfortunately, explanations did not help.

As she lay dying less than three months later, I asked our young pastor to call on her in the hospital to see if she had any spiritual issues she wanted to discuss. She took his hand as he talked to her. *"Oh, you are a good boy,"* she said over and over. I knew within myself that she was ready to die.

3. SENSE OF BEAUTY

Mother had a rare sense of beauty. She had always been a lady who carried herself with grace, beauty, and a sense of style. Yet she was never vain or pretentious. Even to her last months, when memory had almost totally failed her, she seemed to know what was beautiful. Her love of beauty had been evidenced throughout her whole life. Her home, even in the midst of poverty, had spots of beauty with wallpaper, homemade quilts, and various inexpensive crafts. In her garden she had combined the practical needs of her family with areas of intense beauty of flowers. She tended them as if they were truly friends. As the family's poverty decreased, mother took up various forms of art—textile, oil, and china painting. She was a cake decorator. Many a bride was able to say that her wedding had been graced by a fruit cake decorated (and perhaps even baked) by her. Mother decorated my wedding cake, but the most memorable of all her decorated wedding cakes belonged to my niece, Linda. Linda was my sister Joyce's daughter and lived in Manitoba. Mom baked and decorated her cake. It had three layers, and was very ornate. Martin and I drove Mother and the cake from British Columbia to Manitoba for her wedding. The cake arrived in good condition, much to the delight of Linda and her family.

Right up to the last months of her life my mother loved flowers. She liked African violets and I tried to ensure that she had one in full bloom in a pot, placed where she could enjoy it. In winter I bought her books with beautiful pictures of roses. Most of the time she enjoyed looking at them, but sometimes she would say with puzzlement, *"But I can't do anything with them."*

4. PICKING FRUIT

The day was dark and dingy. Autumn had crept into our lives, stripping the vines and trees of all their fruit. I watched as mother walked out the door and went outside. As she walked around the yard, I noticed that she was examining each bush and tree. I knew what she was looking for—it was fruit. All her life she had picked fruit—as a child in Manitoba—as a farmer outside of Vernon—even here on our farm she picked fruit. Mother loved nature of all kinds. The little Vernon farm over-looked a peaceful lake, and under my parents' care it came alive. Flowers, shrubs, fruit trees, and garden produce all flourished.

In her earlier years of dementia she spent hours out in the sunshine, which she loved, picking the strawberries that grew in the raised bed Tony had built for her. Now in later stages of the illness, there remained dim memories of that which she loved to do.

I think of all persons with Alzheimer's and wonder if some of their restless wandering is related to a loved but almost forgotten activity.

5. THE POWER OF A SONG

Mother had slipped into a depressed state of mind. Oh, we tried our best to take her out and do things that interested her but it was getting harder each day.

One night when my sister Joyce and her husband Roy were visiting, I invited some friends in for a night of song. Roy is a guitar player and a lover of music. One of our guests was a banjo player, and we all loved to sing. Mother joined us, although it was her usual bedtime. She became animated with joy, clapping her hands and tapping her knees. It was almost rapturous to watch her. For a time she forgot her confusion and restlessness—she had found her element of joy.

Mom's father was of Irish descent; maybe that's where her love of lively music and rhythm arose. As her dementia increased I often put on an audiotape of Celtic music. Every time, she became alive with joy and I realized the power of a song.

6. MOM AND THE CHILDREN

Through the years as Mom's mental and physical health were declining, there always remained the essence of who she was and always had been. Mother had always been gentle and kind and beneath all her problems she was still the same person.

She had always loved children. Even in church young children gathered around her. She particularly loved one young girl who always seemed to be caring for some other young children. She often said to me, *"That girl is a good girl."* There were many others who came to sit on her knee or just be near her, and she loved them all.

One day three of her granddaughters came to visit her. They were very kind and loving. When they left she said, *"What lovely girls!"* Her daughter answered, "Mom, they are your grandchildren." *"Well, I don't know who they are, but they were lovely,"* sincerely responded Mother.

Some of my most vivid memories are of Mom's interactions with my two youngest grandchildren, Sarina and Morgan. She had been close to them since their births and they often visited her. She was always cold and needed extra blankets to cover her when she was sitting down. Lovingly the little girls would bring a blanket and tuck it all around her. Mom always referred to them as the "little ones" and looked forward to their visits.

Occasionally the 'little ones' would tire Mom. One night as I tucked her into bed she said, *"Where are the little ones?"* "They have gone home, Mom," I responded. *"Good!"* Mom said. "Oh Mom, I thought you liked the little ones." *"Oh, I do,"* Mother said, *"but they are so wild."* Nevertheless, she adored the children and looked forward to their visits. Frequently mother asked if there was enough food for the children, or did they need to sleep with her.

Mother's love and concern for children was always evident, even during the most depressing moments. The 'little ones' had not been at our place for two days. Even though she was resting she said, *"I should get up and see where the kiddies are."* One night as she was just about to fall asleep she opened her eyes and said, *"Goodnight. The girls are so cute."* Then she shut her *eyes and went to sleep. (Journal, Jan. 28/98)* During her last days in the hospital, she asked over and over about the "little ones". Her lifetime habit and concern carried through right to the very end.

She had one Home Support worker who was very petite. I think Mom must have thought she was a child. Mother often told her to say hello to her mother. One day when this particular worker came, she asked mother if she remembered her. Mom laughed and said, *"I remember you when you were like this,"* and she swayed back and forth with arms outspread as if rocking a little baby. The worker had come as an adult from the Philippines and there was no way my mother could have known her as a child. Of course, she thought she did and enjoyed the perception. The worker wisely laughed and did not correct her.

October 26, 1997: Jim, Ginny, and children came Thursday night—left yesterday a.m. Mother enjoyed everyone, and was upset when they went home. Saturday morning, prior to their departure, she woke up and said, "I've been looking for the children, and I told her they were sleeping." She said, "Well, I'd like them right in my room where I can see them."

7. CARING

All her life my mother seemed to embody caring and compassion. As a child she was the second born and the first girl of the second family of her father. The family increased at a fast rate. Mom became the second mother to her many siblings. As each child came, she was kept out of school to look after the children. I have often thought that my mother must have been innately intelligent. She displayed many incredible abilities, yet only achieved a grade eight education.

In her final illness as she lay in a near-coma state, her concentration was on the other three women in the ward with her. I was told that at one time, she even tried to get out of bed so that she could help one of them. Because of her Alzheimer's disease, Mother always had one of her family or a paid attendant with her, and she would instruct us to go and help first one and then another of these women. Her love always shone through.

8. HUMOUR

Mother had always been fun loving and humorous in a quiet, gentle way. One day she very earnestly said to me, "Where is your mother?" I said, "You are my mother. Haven't I got a good mother?" She laughed and said, "You sure have!"

I always felt guilty when I laughed at something funny she had done, because it was so sad. Yet when we laughed together there was something joyous about it. Sometimes it was hard to tell whether she was being funny or just lacked the ability to express herself. One night I was assisting Mom into bed she said, "*But what will I do with my feet?*" I smilingly replied, "I think we'll keep them with you." She laughed, " *Well, I hope so.*" Those were precious and fun moments with her, which reminded me of her essential nature: pleasant and humorous.

One day a visitor said to us, "When you get old you get to know all the bones in your body because they all ache." Mom replied, *"I'm not old enough yet."* In truth she was twenty to thirty years older than the rest of us.

Another night Mother was very tired. She said, *"I don't know why I'm so tired."* I said, *"Well, you are getting older."* She laughed: *"Getting! I've gotten!"* (Strange how sometimes she could express herself in a more typical and complex way.)

Here are some other episodes from my journal:

June 28, 1997: Still a little humour. This a.m. after bath I asked her if she wanted to lie on top of the bed. She said, "I'd like to lie under the bed." Then she laughed at herself—even though I could see she was discouraged and somewhat depressed.

January 19, 1998: When I helped her out of her chair tonight, we both had a laughing fit. She was helping to get up by pushing her hands on the arms of her chair. I was helping with the 'bum lift'. One of my hands was under her bottom and one under her arm. She still wasn't moving, and we both laughed and laughed. When we settled down we tried again and were successful. She went to bed in a good mood. Occasionally, in the evenings when she was tired and trying to get up from her chair she would say, "I don't know if I can get up, I'm sitting on myself."

January 28, 1998: Showing a lot of humour. Good mood. Sat on commode (with seat down) and held pillows while the Home Support person changed her bed. She drummed on pillows and when the Home Support worker leaned over, she drummed on her behind. She thought it was hilarious. Even though it was inappropriate!

Treasures of Life:
Precious Memories of a Precious Mother

PART FOUR
CAREGIVING

1. SHARING THE EXPERIENCE

I remember how I longed for someone with whom to communicate—someone who had similar experiences. Now I am talking to you through written words so that you might know that many of our experiences are jointly owned.

If you were to ask me what my greatest lessons were, I guess I would say there were only a few.

One is to forget what you believe to be true and go with the person's perceptions. This avoids the accumulation of resentment and aggression. It also helps you understand why the person is responding in a certain way.

The second is to understand that even though you have solved a problem today, you may have to solve it again tomorrow. Problems quickly change in complexity. You will most likely have to adjust the solution very soon because of the gradual deterioration in cognition and memory.

The third, and most important, is to always display gentleness, kindness, and love. That may not be easy, but nothing truly worthwhile is ever easy.

2. WONDERFUL SUPPORT

When mother first came to live with us four years before her death, I was working full time. Because she was still fairly competent and responsible, I made a deal with her. I would not charge her board and room, but with that money we would hire someone to do something special with her everyday. At first it was mainly to enhance her life, and she and her companion went to special events that Mom was interested in; such as, seniors teas and luncheons, Bible studies, lunches at the restaurant, or just out for pie and coffee.

As time went by, Mother needed extra help. In addition to her companion, we took advantage of the Health Home Support program, especially for bathing and personal care.

Sometimes support came from unexpected sources. A nurse who worked twelve-hour shifts in the hospital offered to come and sit with Mom in her spare time. Although I never called upon her, it still warms my heart to think of her willingness. Another friend of mine, also a nurse, one day surprised us with a visit as Mom and I sat in the yard. I'll never forget her tenderness as she went to Mom, took her hands, looked deep into her eyes, and asked, "How are you, Mrs. Pouncy?" She displayed such a depth of compassion and understanding! Then there was the time when Mother fell and broke her hip. I was sitting outside her room in the hospital as the personnel worked with her. Our pastor's wife came, put her arms around me, and said with compassion: "This was not part of your plan, was it?" How much all the kindness meant I cannot express! Oh, there was also the time when a good friend came and whisked me away for a lunch in a nearby café. How little people understand that one doesn't need to say eloquent words, or to do outstanding deeds to show kindness. Often all that is needed is a few simple words sincerely spoken, an arm around the shoulder, or even a firm handshake. It's the human contact that matters—that speaks volumes.

As my mother's disease progressed, she needed full-time care and I quit my job. I never regretted my decision. Although I was of retirement age, I missed my work. It had filled an important role in my life. It was a sacrifice I was willing to make, and I determined to enhance each day of my mother's life. We had the same amount of help as before because twenty-four hour care is too much for one person to do every day. Sometimes it was very hard, and I had to tell myself over and over again, "Focus. Refocus. Now Focus again."

3. A TEAM EFFORT

Successful caregiving should be a team effort. There is a delicate balance between professionals, other caregivers, family, and the primary caregiver. (In Mother's case that was myself.)

I found my mother's doctors and the local pharmacists to be very competent, supportive, and helpful. They were an important part of an excellent team of care. This was also true of the government Home Care workers and privately hired caregivers. Perhaps integral to all the efforts were those of my family and circle of friends. They provided valuable insights and support.

As the primary caregiver I never expected thanks, but I did expect respect as the person who carried the heaviest load. I expected and experienced people who did their best in whatever role they played.

4. RESPECT AND DIGNITY

Each person in our extended family displayed great respect and love for Mother. This was invaluable. My desire is that other families would demonstrate the same. Yet in society as a whole I note some disrespect for the elderly—indeed for all things old. Of course, generalities never are accurate in all cases, and I have also seen great respect. However, we tend to be in an era of disposable things. If our TV breaks down, it is easier and more economical to buy a new one than to repair the old. Computers are outdated almost as soon as they are marketed.

When we come to human beings, we must recognize the absolute worth of each person. In some societies the elderly are respected not only for the life they gave us but also for their accumulation of knowledge and wisdom. In Alzheimer's disease, knowledge and wisdom gradually seep away, but the person is still a priceless human being, worthy of great respect and dignity.

5. THINKING COMPONENT

I found there was a strong thinking component required in caring for my mother. I was continually questioning and searching for answers: Why was this particular thing (or behaviour) happening? Is there any way I can alleviate her fear, confusion, or anger? How does my mother feel about this situation? What meaning does she see in her life? How can I enhance her life?

I was constantly solving problems. Certainly, I was not always successful; however, I feel certain that my search helped to make her life happier. It also gave me focus and a continual challenge. Incidentally, it is much better to think in terms of challenges instead of problems—to concentrate on the joys instead of on the sorrows and losses.

6. DEVELOPMENT VERSUS MAINTENANCE

Most caregivers of Alzheimer's patients are parents themselves. I had given birth to four children and had gone through years of trying to help my children in their development. As parents we are always thinking of the future. We visualize the men and women that we hope our children will become someday. We hope they will have skills that will enable them to find employment and to lead meaningful and useful lives. This is certainly not the case with Alzheimer's disease. The individuals are losing skills, not gaining them.

Although adults with Alzheimer's disease may have some child-like behaviours, they are not children. Our task in their care is not to develop their abilities or even to maintain them. Instead it is that of giving meaning to each day, to relieve the negative effects of the disease as far as possible, and to bring a measure of peace and enjoyment to our loved one. It is better to lay aside our child-rearing skills and expectations.

7. EASY OR HARD?

If I make it sound easy to have served a beloved mother when she had Alzheimer's disease that is not my intention. It was hard—very hard. Only great love and perseverance did the job. Nor is it my intention to discourage anyone. There were also many great rewards that I would have missed had I chosen a different path.

It is difficult to explain why the job was so hard. Perhaps the constant worry and concern. When I went to bed it was only to sleep lightly, and I was frequently up to tend her. Often mother would be restless at night. We ensured her safety by turning off the stove breaker at night, and latching the basement door. Outside doors were dead-bolted and she could not open them. Even so when I heard her, I got up to see how I could help her. Sometimes Martin relieved me. I tucked her into bed, and if she was extremely disturbed, I tried to sleep in an easy chair in her room. During one period of her illness, I even slept on a mat in her room—gradually moving out as she improved. The occasional night she slept through. That was so unusual that I thought she must have died in her sleep. Either way I suffered from lack of sleep. I had to contend daily with my constant tiredness. Sometimes I would take a little nap in the daytime, but mother never really liked that. She appreciated hard-working people, not people she perceived as lazy!

Another very human difficulty was to always put my mother before my own needs. Martin rarely made a comment on my dedication to her, but on one occasion he did. "Your life is centered entirely around your mother." I told him that I would concentrate on any family member who was ill and in trouble. Fortunately for me, I have a very understanding husband. I somehow managed to feed Martin and the rest of my family when they came to visit—somehow I coped, in retrospect I'm not sure how I did it all. The risk in caregiving is to neglect your own needs, and perhaps I did that at times.

November 16, 1997: Find myself at the end of second consecutive day of constant attention, with my patience wearing a little thin. Mom ate a large, late lunch; had a banana snack at four p.m. Now at four forty-five (she is) looking for supper. It's constant and unremitting. I'm grateful for the opportunity to serve. It is with love that I serve. May God give me patience sixty minutes an hour; twenty-four hours per day; 365 days per year. I know it is much worse for her—she lives with something she cannot understand, the same number of minutes a year. She does extremely well. May God grant her peace.

We had many helpers that greatly eased the load. The hard part associated with that is that every person had an opinion as to how I might physically care for Mom. I had to constantly insist on relying on the medical professionals—her doctor and the pharmacists. I recognize the good intentions, but now and then mental pressures built up that made the job harder than it needed to be. I was so happy that my family totally trusted me and did not question my judgment. An entry in my journal will demonstrate how I felt at the time:

February 7, 1998: The more serious the situation, the less I appreciate theories and advice. I want to work directly with the doctor and pharmacist. It's amazing how much advice I get—from people with good intentions. It's like an additional assault on my mind, although I dearly appreciate and love the caring people.

What the doctors and I have to constantly do is balance the good and life-saving effects of the drugs with the negative effects that in themselves may endanger health. That's one reason I want the doctor to take the ultimate responsibility, although I certainly want my input. I feel certain within myself that our efforts have given Mom a fair amount of extra time with us already.

Overall, the good far outweighed the negative. It was my great privilege to care for my mother. I feel so fortunate to have had that opportunity and to have had wonderful people helping in the difficult job.

8. FOCUSING

Because caregiving was constant, it was very intense and tiring. I have learned through my life that goal-setting is a vital skill in all phases of life. It was particularly helpful in caregiving. My goal and purpose was to enhance each day of Mother's life. To do that, I had to focus. That was not always easy, but without it I do not believe her life would have been nearly as happy in the last few years. A couple of illustrations from my journal will demonstrate this point:

June 28, 1997: Mom not at all well. My heart goes out to her in love. Something is changing in her body. I must be strong for her and all.

Focus~~~Love.

Refocus~~~Love

& Focus Again~~~Love.

July 8, 1997: I must constantly FOCUS—REFOCUS— and FOCUS AGAIN on my positive goals. Sometimes weariness takes over and I lose my vision.

9. OBSERVING HER DISTRESS

The motivation for caring for a beloved mother is great love, without that love twenty-hour caregiving would be just too difficult. This strong love is also the reason the stress is also so intense. It is very difficult to daily observe the tension, fear, and distress that your loved one is experiencing.

One night Mother was very tense. I comforted her the best I could but she never relaxed. She would shut her eyes and periodically open them. At one point she had her hands and arms in the air and she motioned, as if she were feeling or searching for something. I asked her, "Are you in pain? Does it hurt anywhere?" She answered, *"No, I am just lost...lost."* I stayed with her throughout the evening and until about 20 minutes to 3 a.m., when she at last gave me permission to go to bed. My comments in my journal at that time said this: *I can't imagine what 'hell' it would be for her, if she had a caregiver who was impatient and unsympathetic. My heart aches for her.*

December 5, 1997: Mom seems quiet but unhappy. When I asked her she said, "There's nothing for me." I said, "You went to town to Wayne's (her hairdresser) and got your hair done. You got a lovely card from Frank and Joan." She forgets as soon as she does something so thinks she has done nothing. My journal reveals my stress when I wrote: *"It is hard to see her unhappy, espe-*

cially when she is imagining things and there's nothing I can do to fix it."

10. LITTLE THINGS

Important events and the inevitable downhill path certainly cause stress as you watch the health of your loved one deteriorate; yet little things can also cause stress. For example, one week was exceptionally emotional and I was tired. It was early in the evening and there was a good movie on the television. I had just settled down to watch it and she wanted to go to bed. I gave her some soup and crackers to eat and then got her ready for bed. Once more I started to watch the movie, but it was just a few minutes and she was out again. Forget the movie, Gerry—you are a caregiver. Although 99.99% of the time I was patient, I felt just a touch of frustration. I'm sure that happens in all cases of caregiving when it is a full-time job. Here is an excerpt from my journal:

Feel some stress. Must take steps so do not burn out. I have been very busy lately. Mom restless and agitated today. I sat with her as supper was cooking and she settled down.

11. TIREDNESS

Perhaps my biggest hazard was the tiredness that was ever present. Of course, I've mentioned it many times before, but it underlay all my personal problems. As you read through the pages of this book. I'm sure you can understand why that was the case. The following journal entries are tiny samples of the constant state of tiredness that I experienced.

September 30: 1997: Myself: Very tired. Stress helped by visitors, but tiredness escalated. Personal control (is) very important. It's hard to stay calm, restful, and stress-free, with the constant attentiveness and putting off (of my) own needs. Yet I have an important personal goal: "To enhance each day of Mom's life."

December 7, 1997: I seem to be feeling better. I was so tired (that I) had trouble functioning.

December 19, 1997: Off to bed for me. I must keep my health and emotional equilibrium. This is a vicious illness. She is still my very precious mother. I do not ask why—although it would be an easy question to ask.

I have been editing this book, hoping to soon send it to the publishers (August 27, 2004). Today I took my ten-year-old granddaughter, Sarina, out for what we call Grandma Day. I was telling her about my book and about Mom's sleeping problems. She knows a person with Alzheimer's and she said very knowingly: "Oh, she doesn't have any problems with sleep—no problems at all. Her problems are when she's awake, not when she's asleep." I laughed and laughed. Of course she is right. Mom's problems and incidentally mine, were not when she was asleep! Humour is a great healer and even in retrospect I enjoy a great joke about the situation.

12. COPING

Caregiving is very difficult. Many caregivers go into periods of depression. Because of my prior knowledge, I knew of the dangers and tried to take whatever precautions possible. I went to a workshop on caregiving. It was excellent. Yet strangely, I just wanted to cry—I almost never shed tears!

I started a communications log. At first Mother was able to read and comprehend some of it. When Mom could no longer comprehend it, the log was used to inform workers and other members of my family about the activities and problems of the day.

Then I started a journal that I shared with other workers. When one worker started to make comments about my recorded feelings, I decided the journals were for me alone. Just to write down daily happenings helped to put them into some kind of perspective and chart the course of Mom's illness. They also proved therapeutic for me. It is from these journals that I have written the excerpts in this book.

A couple of months before Mom's death, the Home Support supervisor noticed that I was under stress. She offered to get funding for a worker to care for Mom one evening each week. Gratefully, my husband and I chose it as our date-night. Often my mother did not like me going out, but I realized that to be a good caregiver I needed to care for myself.

Our children and other family members were tremendously supportive to us. In addition, the people of our church sustained our spirits by caring and praying. Without support I'm not sure how a person would be able to cope. It certainly made a tremendous difference in my life, and of course in the life of my lovely mother.

13. JOURNAL ENTRIES

As I write these stories six years after Mom's death, I reread my journals. They were such a help to me as I went through the difficult times. I find quotes like this one:

Mom is so very mixed up. I thank God for the ability he has given me to calm her down. It is so very difficult for her.

Mom up again. Is mentioning Dad. "Have you seen

Dad?" I tell her about Dad's death and soon after she questions again. "Have you seen Dad? Is he around? Tell him..." (and her voice trailed off) I responded to her, "You rest now, Mom. We will talk about it in the morning."

Constantly she is mixed up, confused, and agitated. I understand; how would I feel if the past were all muddled up and incomprehensible. It's somewhat like being in a nightmare all the time. But it's hard for me too. I care so much and am so emotionally involved. How can I keep my sanity? It's hard.

Another quote says: *Suffering a bit of burn out. Too many responsibilities. Yet I know that looking at the problems instead of the possibilities is counterproductive. I constantly tell myself to Focus, Refocus, and Focus again. That is my motto as well as another, "This day I will enhance my mother's life."* Those days were very difficult ones. Would I do it again if the need arose and I was able? Yes, a thousand times, yes. She usually did not recognize me as her daughter, but to see her eyes light up with loving recognition was compensation enough, as well as to know that I had done my very best to ease her situation. I was someone who loved and cared for her, and she knew that.

Mom not well at all. Something is changing in her body. I must be strong for her, and (for) all.

Mom some better today.

Back and forth her health zigzagged. Sometimes she seemed to be dying and other days she made amazing recoveries—although the memory loss was quite consistent. It was not the only problem though. Some of her problems were of a very personal nature and very disturbing. I studied my Merck's medical manual and parked on the doctor and pharmacist's doorsteps, taking advantage of all their knowledge and wisdom.

14. TO LAUGH OR NOT TO LAUGH

To laugh or not to laugh, that is the question. It should be easy to answer, but when someone you love has Alzheimer's there is no simple answer to the dilemma.

My mom and dad were married for 62 years. One day at a family reunion when Mother was in the beginning stages of her disease, family members were talking at the camp where we met. Someone mentioned that Mom and Dad had been married. With great dignity and strong emotion Mother said, *"Harry Pouncy! I never married Harry Pouncy! I would never marry Harry Pouncy!"* Everyone burst into laugher, not fully realizing how fragile mother's memory was, and how her tiredness was promoting its loss.

Another time, I was in our kitchen when Mom came to me holding a capped Bic pen. *"I don't know how to work this," she said. I demonstrated how to take off the cap and gave it back. At that she began to use the pen on her face as if it were a razor. I started to laugh. Then I realized how very sad it really was, and I turned away so she could not see my tears. The dilemma is that in order to work lovingly and long with someone with serious memory loss you must retain your sense of humor. At the same time it is necessary to maintain the dignity of the person you serve, and respect her at all times. That is not an easy balance.*

I remember one evening when Mom was quite upset. She said (referring to her Home Care worker), "She told someone I was shaky. I am not shaky." With that she twirled around. "See," she said, "my pants aren't falling off." With that we both started to laugh. "Oh, Mom", I said, "I'm so glad you haven't lost your sense of humour".

She replied, "Well, it's better to laugh than to cry—isn't it?"

One day my teen-age grandson Andrew and I decided to take Mom to the café for a piece of pie and a cup of tea. It was a wonderful time of togetherness for all three of us.

Mom sat there looking at her surroundings. A sign had been placed on the piano: "No smoking, please." Mom turned to me and said, *"Would you like a smoke?"* Andrew and I burst into laughter for I had never smoked in my whole life. Sometimes laughter just tumbled out unplanned, and afterward I wondered how my mother had felt at our response. She never seemed to take offense.

September 30, 1997: At dinner time the other night she was fussing about the food; putting cranberry sauce on the platter of turkey; worrying about food: "Did she have some? Did others have food?" I said, "Everybody has everything. Everyone is looked after." Emphatically Mother picked up her teacup and put it upside down, "What is this then?" I left the room nearly hysterical— not knowing whether to laugh or cry.

15. GENTLING

Gentling's Beginnings

I didn't call it "gentling" until Mom's final years, but I practiced it daily. The word seemed to perfectly describe the process of quieting Mom. Gentling probably started when my little Billy, who was suffering from leukemia, was in his final week. He was in hospital, when suddenly he went blind. He did not have very long to live so I thought there was no reason for him to know the brutal truth. "Turn the lights on, Mommy," he said to me one bright November day.

"Oh, you will sleep better in the dark," I replied. Not a lie, but an evasion of stark reality.

My next significant gentling experience came about twenty-five years later. Martin's mother had come to spend her last years with us. She did not have Alzheimer's disease, but occasionally suffered from a dependency issue. If she did not receive her mild tranquilizer at precisely seven p.m., she had what could be described as a manic attack.

One night I arrived home after working late. My mother-in-law was in a wild, agitated state. I can still see her in my mind. There she stood at the phone in the hall. She wore her outdoor coat and had tied a kerchief around her head. She was trying to phone someone (she had no idea who) to come and take her home—she had momentarily forgotten that she lived with us. Everyone was trying to reason with her, but she would have none of that nonsense!

I went to her and put my arms around her. Tenderly I said, "Oh, Grandma, I have arranged for you to sleep here tonight. You can sleep in this bed." Gently I showed her the bed she slept in every night.

"Oh, thank you, Gerry," she said with grateful emotion.

Momentarily I felt like a dishonest person. It felt slightly like a lie, but in truth I had arranged to have her live with us. Working within the person's perceptions initially was a problem for me because I always tried to strictly adhere to the truth. In order to "gentle a person" it is absolutely necessary to communicate within the person's comprehension, and I had to come to terms with my personal values.

My Helpful Background

I had an advantage over many other caregivers because of my many years' experience working in an organization that served adults with developmental disabilities. Over many years, I learned everything I could about various conditions. I read. I went to multiple workshops, training courses, and conferences. Ultimately I became a manager, and a part-time instructor at a local college. This education and experience was extremely helpful when it came time for me to serve my beloved mother.

Our organization did not punish or belittle our clients but used positive reinforcement with numerous words of encouragement and praise for work well done. The people we served thrived. Miracles happened constantly. I became an absolute believer in the powerful, positive, and gentle approach—not as an act but as a manner of thinking and being. If our gentleness is merely a pretense to serve our purposes, people will detect it. Respect and gentleness must be real.

I am in no way implying that it takes my type of experience and background to care for your loved one. I believe that love can accomplish miracles. I am writing this book to encourage others to couple love with a respectful attitude and an acceptance of the importance of each person they are planning to help.

Gentling my Precious Mother

Mom couldn't understand what was happening to her. Her memory was going bit by bit. She fought it but finally gave up the useless struggle. Everything was strange; everything was frightening. People whom she knew so well became strangers—sometimes nice, but more often they proved menacing. Everyday occurrences became strange and hard to understand. She, who had so often comforted me when I was a child, now needed comforting herself. Another one of my goals became "To Gentle my Mother."

June 9, 1997: Mom so very mixed up. I thank God for the ability he has given me to calm her down. It is so very difficult for her. May God continue to give me the very words to say that will effect peace.

The task that I laid out for myself was not an easy one, but in retrospect it kept me on track. I pulled the drapes at night, when evening shadows became menacing. I gave her a cup of tea when she declared emphatically that she had not eaten a bite all day; of course I knew that she had. What did it matter? What she believed was her reality and as far as possible I reached into her reality and responded to it. If the pressure became heavy, I took a quick time-out and came back with a smile. Mother's mental health depended on my composure and gentle nature.

There's a common saying, "What goes around, comes around," and out of it all I became a gentler more compassionate human being. If my mother knew, I think she would have been pleased. Somewhere in heaven perhaps she is smiling her gentle, sweet smile.

My Piano Playing

My piano playing is extremely amateurish. I took a year or two of lessons when I was a child over sixty years ago. Then I took lessons for a few months when I was almost sixty. You can imagine how bumbling I was on a piano—I was then almost seventy years old!

One day when Mom was sitting beside me I started playing some simple old songs. Mother loved it. As her dementia worsened, I found that she became very agitated and confused late in the afternoon and early evening. So, often I sat down and played a few old songs and she would totally relax. When possible that became a nightly ritual. Often she would clap and attempt to keep time to my offbeat music. Other times she would nod off to sleep. When I stopped she usually woke, but she was relaxed, and would remain so throughout her bedtime ritual.

Redirecting

Experience is a great teacher. I learned to divert attention from situations that most likely would result in misunderstandings.

One day Mom brought out her favourite black sweater with colourful flowers on it. She gave it to me as a gift. "Thanks, Mom," I said, "we'll just put it over this chair. If I need it, I will wear it. If you need it, you can wear it". Mother seemed very grateful. That response was much more successful than, "That's your sweater, Mom, you wear it." It was important to accept her gift while not really taking it. She always wanted to be generous.

Another night Mother talked of getting her coat and going home. I said, "Everything is in your room. Here is your supper." After supper she still was determined to get her things so that she could go home. So I said to her, "Come to your bedroom. I will help you." In the bedroom I directed her to her commode. Then we got her clothes off and her nightgown on, and I helped her into bed. She had forgotten about going home.

November 15, 1997: Mother very restless. She is going over and over things, trying to make sense of her world, I guess. As a caregiver it tends to be a little wearing and depressing. There is no discrimination as to ownership. This morning she went around gathering things up. "I'm deciding what I want and don't want." She asked for her books. I spread them out on the table thinking she wanted to look them over, but no. She piled them all up in about three or four piles along with her purse and some other things (pictures, etc.). Then she asked me for something to put them in. I have a notion she may have been thinking of 'going' and deciding on what to take. I redirected and took her into town for lunch. Of course, I quietly put the things away.

January 12, 1998: Mom restless and 'cranky'. She is looking at the rose book. "I can't see how I could ever do this." She counted the roses. "What can you do with them?" Yesterday she said, "Aren't they beautiful? Gorgeous!" Today: "Oh, I can't do anything. I am stupid." Why the change in reactions? It's hard to predict. I'm trying to turn it around: "It's (rose) beautiful," etc. Guess I'll go and get a snack for her and break the cycle.

One night she was obsessing over the name of someone whose picture she saw. We told her his name was David. *"No,"* she said, *"it isn't."* She was trying very hard to remember. Finally I said, "Would you like me to put the picture up, and we'll try to think of his name?" She agreed, very relieved at the solution. It was the end of the subject (out of sight; out of mind).

Gentling and Acceptance

To be able to gentle a person with dementia it is necessary that we totally accept the person—not only to accept the person but the place that person is in their life cycle.

It is important to help the person in ways that maintain his (or her) dignity in the community. This involves the way we assist in personal care and the manner in which we address him. Talk to him, not just to the person accompanying him.

Involve the person with appropriate tasks and choices. They should never be beyond his ability to achieve. To offer gentle and respectful help is appropriate. Gently asking if you can help ensures that the person has the choice to accept or reject your offer.

Night Gentling

Usually mornings were relatively restful for Mother. Problems arose as the day progressed into late afternoon, evening, and night. Restlessness, confusion, disorientation, paranoia, and other disturbing conditions became common. So often Home Care workers and her companion were gone before the problems became intense.

When I tucked her into bed, I would tell her that I loved her and would take care of everything. She was not to worry. Sometimes that was all the reassurance that she needed.

Other times it was not that easy. One night Martin and I planned to go out for our weekly date. A home care worker was overseeing Mom. Mother was not happy. She stated, *"I don't like this place. I am going to kill myself and go to hell. Don't expect me to live. I am going to go home."* Gently I led her to her bedroom. "Here Mom, I will help you." I got her ready for bed, even though it was only 5:30 p.m., and rubbed her back. I told her I loved her; gave her a mild sedative, and tucked her into bed with a 'warm bag' placed beside her cheek. After fixing the light to her specifications, I kissed her again and said goodnight. At that she settled down and slept through until 3:30 a.m. When I went to her, she had a tear in her eye. She said, *"I was looking and looking for you, and I couldn't find you."* She was very loving. It is very important that you do not take offense at any anger or negative statements directed at you. The anger is really at her memory loss and total confusion. Always respond with love and gentleness. Taking extra time to comfort and to quiet your loved one pays huge dividends. It not only brings peace to your loved one but reduces the anger and agitation that would ultimately cause serious problems.

Sometimes I thought that going out was hardly worth

the trouble, but I always came back to the fact that caregivers really do have to care for themselves so they can be loving and kind to the persons they look after.

Go with the Flow

It is essential to gentling, that the caregiver goes with the flow. This only makes sense, but it is often hard to do. Often caregivers bring past problems to the present relationship and may say or think things like: "She has often been difficult, I remember when...." At the point a story may emerge. It most likely will be of some disagreement that had happened some years previously. It is important to drop all past grievances and work only on the present with gentleness and tenderness. To go against the person, their misperceptions, or lack of reality is only to invite trouble. The absolute truth is no matter how you try, you cannot change your loved one's behaviour except by love, gentleness, respect and acceptance. He or she no longer has the ability to conceptualize the positive changes needed to make the relationship more positive. The caregiver must do that.

> *It is absolutely essential that each person be treated with dignity and respect*

PART FIVE

PRECIOUS MEMORIES

1. GOOD FOR EVERYTHING

One day I was doing some little task for Mom. She said, "Oh, you are good for everything." I teasingly responded, "Mom, I'm glad you didn't say, 'I'm good for nothing'". Mother laughed and lovingly said, "Oh, I would never say that".

Mother had been very restless all day. That night I tucked her into bed several times. During the night, I came down to her one more time. She said, "I called and called you and I couldn't get you, but now you kissed me and everything is O.K."

Oh, what precious memories flood me of my very loving mother. Although there were many difficult times in her illness, I determined that I would treasure each moment and every shared laugh. That I've always done!

Sometimes there was a sweet, childlike reliance on me. One day she insisted on being with me. *"I have known Gerry for a long time."* Later I invited her to sit with me on the love seat. She said, *"Just you and me— no one else."* I held her hand and she really liked that. *(Journal, December 9, 1997)*

2. HER FINAL BIRTHDAY

The morning of her birthday celebration dawned but Mom was not feeling well; however, by the afternoon when her celebrations were planned she was better. She thoroughly enjoyed opening her presents, and enjoyed the family who had gathered around her in love. She almost appeared like her pre-disease self. Of course, it only lasted for a short time, but every moment of joy was a precious memory.

It is worth noting that even though the quiet life was soothing, family was vitally important to Mother. The impact of loving family members circling both her, and Martin and me, was priceless.

3. HER FINAL CHRISTMAS

Christmas morning came and my mother had no idea what was going on. We opened our gifts while she had her daily bath. I could tell that the Home Support worker did not understand this decision but we knew that Mother would be totally confused with the excitement—the quiet life agreed with her better. Our children and grandchildren had come to celebrate with us and it was a very busy time.

I had arranged with my daughters-in-law to cook, serve the dinner, and clean up while I stayed in the bedroom with Mom. It was a special time although it was also stressful.

After dinner, Mother sat in the easy chair in our living room, while our son Jim started tossing balloons around. Mom got into the action, throwing the balloons back and forth to him and other family members. It was one of those exceptional and treasured memories. For a short period of time, she became animated and a picture of health and vitality.

These incidents and all the memories are precious and fill my storehouse of love. Each day was a gift to celebrate and cherish.

4. TIDBITS OF LOVE

There are not many rewards in giving care to a person with severe memory loss, but the few are extremely precious. One day Mother said to me, "I've been looking and looking for you, to see that you're O.K. I replied, "Well, I am here and I'm O.K." She said, "I can see that, and I love you." Did she think I was her mother or was I her daughter Gerry at that moment? I don't know and it really doesn't matter. She loved me.

Another evening Mom seemed very tired, but each time I asked her if she wanted to go to bed she said, *"No, I just want to look at you!"* Did she realize how precious time was and was she storing up love? I don't know.

December 20, 1997: Sweet this early a.m. I lovingly tucked her in and she said, "Her is kind," and she added quizzically, "I think...?"

January 6, 1998: Mom up after 3 a.m.; I got up at 3:45. Got her back to bed and covered her up. She firmly and kindly said, "You are a good woman." She repeated it. I said, "You are a good woman too." With that she smiled and settled down.

January 10, 1998: Mom now in bed 9:15 p.m. Up since lunch. Hope she sleeps tonight. Every night when I tuck her in, I tuck a' warm bag' by her cheek, kiss her and say, "I love you." She responds, "I love you too". Precious words. Others may see all the difficulties, and of course I see them too, but I also see and experience the love.

January 20, 1998: Mom thanked Martin for the fire he made in the fireplace and all the nice things he does...I was helping Mom today and she said, "You are good to me," with a lot of emphasis. Felt good.

It is an honour to serve a noble purpose—
Caring for a beloved person is such a purpose

PART SIX

FINAL DAYS

1. MY REALIZATION

As Mother's physical and mental health deteriorated, I realized that each day she had with us was a gift. When I tucked her into bed at night, I said goodbye to her in my heart, because I knew time was short and precious. As she greeted me each morning, I was thankful for yet another day with my precious mother. The following is an excerpt from my journal:

November 26, 1997: Bed by 5:30—very weak. Almost like a child. Took pill, "Did I do it right?" Same with spoons of food. Ate several pieces of carrot, one spoon of squash and a taste of applesauce, bit of tea. Very sweet. People are again talking 'end of life'. For a year or two now I have been on a roller coaster. Trying to enhance each day of her life and yet knowing it is not entirely within my hands. God will decide when, not I. I just want to do my best.

My sister, Joyce, lived in Manitoba and could not be with her much, although she did come for an occasional visit. My other sister, Alica, who lived in Sechelt, BC, came as often as possible. In early 1998, she and her husband were planning to go to Hawaii. We arranged that they were to come and see Mother before they left. In truth, it was to be the last time they were to see Mom alive. My brother Frank and his wife planned to go to Arizona for the winter, but visited her before they left. I think they must have mentally said goodbye every time they left her as well. It was obvious that her time on earth was limited. Mother loved each one of her family. She did not know their names or who they were, yet she knew somehow that they were special and that they loved her.

2. MOTHER'S REALIZATION

I think that Mom had some vague idea of death. Although she had forgotten many things, statements she made indicated some knowledge and understanding. The following are some excerpts from my journal:

October 18, 1997: Last night Mom was very tired. She was worried about all the 'things'—indicating the things in the kitchen. I said, "Don't worry tonight. We're tired. Tomorrow we will fix everything up." She said, "I want you and the other kids to get everything." I responded, "I know you've been keeping things for your kids. I'll see that they get them." This is at least the second time she has mentioned this. I think she is realizing that life is coming to an end. She also said, "I know my mother is really worried about me." Interesting, because I am also her mother and I change roles very easily and quickly, and of course I do worry.

November 1, 1997: Mom very tired last night—didn't wake in the evening, as is her custom. (So I didn't give her Oxazapam.) Then (she) woke about 2 a.m.—up and down, up and down. First Martin tried to settle her—success in neighborhood of a few minutes. Then I got up and gave her Oxazapam—not very effective until finally she fell asleep approaching four a.m. On one of my settling attempts she very quietly said, "I can't believe I am still alive." I wasn't sure the first time what she said so she repeated. I said, "Well, you are very old, but you are doing well." She did not seem agitated—just very awake. Although I think when she wakes in the night she always seems a little anxious and often I see a tear in her eye. I am very gentle and tender with her and she thanks me. These will be precious memories someday of my precious Mom.

3. TO LIVE OR TO DIE?

Mother often had her breakfast on a TV tray, while she sat in a comfortable wicker chair. One morning I looked over at her. She looked dead. I spoke to her. She did not answer. I quickly went to her and took her pulse. Her heart was beating but I could not rouse her. My husband went to the phone and called the ambulance while I stayed with her. I continued to try to arouse her. Finally she started to respond, but she was frightened and said, "I am dying. I have never felt this way before. It is awful. I am dying."

Quietly I talked to her. "Mom, what do you want? Do you want to die and go to heaven and be with Jesus, or do you want to live?" She thought for a minute and then said, *"I guess I want to go to heaven."*

About that time my son Tony walked in the back door. The ambulance came with two personnel. Then an RCMP officer came, and lastly a Home Support worker. The female paramedic said, "Oh, I'm glad we didn't have to do CPR." I was horrified that anyone would consider giving CPR to a frail, elderly woman who was obviously nearing the end of her life. The ambulance drove Mother to the hospital and the Home Support worker comforted me. It was a very emotional experience.

4. A SERIOUS DECISION

The day after Mom's episode of unconsciousness, I went to visit her doctor. I told her about the comment of the ambulance attendant. The doctor said, "It would have been their duty to give CPR. To prevent it you would have had to present a Do Not Resuscitate Order." The doctor agreed with me that the procedure would be cruel and unnecessary, and I filled out the form. I kept it handy, but never had to use it. It was something that I had never considered up to that point.

5. THE ACCIDENT

In our minds we constantly said goodbye to Mother, knowing that her time was very limited. I expected that I would come into her room one morning and find that she had died, but how little we know and are able to predict. On February 18, 1998, she fell in our living room. She was obviously in pain and I called the ambulance. She was lying flat on the floor and I tried my best to keep her in that position. I had a pillow at her head, and a blanket over her. She adamantly refused to stay lying down. She could not understand the reason and fought to get up. Finally, I propped some chesterfield pillows behind her, and a folded blanket under her knees. I sat on the floor with her and supported her the best way that I could. The paramedics came, and one of them reprimanded me for not keeping her lying flat—how little others understand the predicament that a caregiver can get into, even though trying to follow the correct procedures.

As soon as she was taken to the hospital, the doctor made the diagnosis of a broken hip. He told me that she needed an operation. "She will not survive an operation," I said. He responded, "She will not survive if she does not have an operation." So I agreed.

She survived the operation, and lived for another two and one-half weeks. That was a precious time, although it was also filled with concern for her welfare. We arranged for twenty-four hour extra care at the hospital—either one of the family or a hired attendant. She was often confused and disoriented and sometimes she fought the necessary procedures, but as she became more comfortable she became calmer.

Eating and drinking became major problems. She had lost all understanding of why they were necessary and she ate and drank very little. In the end that is why she died.

Mother had odd little glimpses of reality and understanding. One day Martin and Tony came in. She was quite lucid when Tony was there (for about one half an hour). When he left she lapsed back into confusion.

I contacted my siblings and told them that Mom was probably dying. Family members and a few friends came to see her. She seemed to be slipping away one day when Tony came in again. From her near-coma state, she opened her eyes and knowingly said, *"Tony, I know you, Tony."* She always had special connections with my sons, who had been so good to her.

When I arrived at the hospital the morning after the operation, she looked at me and said, *"Joyce?"* I said, "No, Gerry." She called me Gerry (not mother) all day. Interesting sometimes that pain seems to bring a type of mental alertness while diminishing other skills—or was it simply the results of impending death. I don't know.

February 19, 1998: Yesterday while waiting in Emergency Department, Mom asked over and over about the little ones, as if she were looking for them. A little child was crying in the next compartment in E.R. Mom was very concerned. She talks a lot about the children she had, but the numbers vary. Her concern is constant.

The days and weeks leading up to her death are somewhat of a blur in my memory; however, I did record some of my feelings at that time:

February 28, 1998: It is a lonely path sitting with Mom. It is also sad. We have lots of company of good people but there's so much empty time. Mom just sleeps and sleeps unless she is in distress.

The nurses and other staff are good. Very busy though. Nurses are overworked—hardly getting time to eat. Mom talked again of dying. A friend asked her if that's what she wants. Mom didn't answer. She does seem to have lost hope and the zest for living.

6. PLANNING FOR MOTHER'S FUTURE

For a while, my mother seemed as if she might survive. Even though a doctor had informed me that I could no longer care for my mother in my home, I schemed and schemed how it might be possible. I asked to speak to a social worker. I told him that I thought I could manage if I had forty hours of Home Support—eight hours a night, which would include her bath, and four hours a week for respite. He informed me that unfortunately the system was not set up to help families to that degree. Hearing his discouraging words I penned the following in my journal: My whole thoughts are on quality of life for her. My goal has been to enhance each day of her life. I am still trying to do that. The methods may change but the principles remain. (February 28, 1998)

7. GOODBYE, EARTH—HELLO, HEAVEN

Finally, less than three weeks after the fall, Mother died. Her body could no longer support her spirit. In death as in her life she displayed love. I lost count of the many times she told me she loved me. It was so sweet and precious—final gifts of love. They were worth the many times of stress and concern. She was my beloved mother, ready to meet her God.

Yet even in those last hours she had mixed perceptions of who she was, and who I was. She often said to me, "Gerry is dying. Gerry is very sick." She had somehow become me, and I had become her. It was strange to me—somehow my identity had almost been lost in hers. I went with her every step of the way to the gates of heaven, but I stayed and she went.

She finally slipped away early morning, while all the hospital was quiet. The nurse on duty was so kind and comforting. She told me Mom had gone and I took Mother's pulse. I found what I believed to be a heart beat and told her. It seemed to me as if she were going very slowly. The hospital staff let Martin and me stay in her room until the doctor arrived later (somewhere around 9 a.m.) and declared death.

Some of our family came to the hospital, and our son Gordie and his wife Karen took us to a café for breakfast on the way home. I felt like I was walking in a dream, as if I were an observer seeing the world anew.

8. HER FUNERAL

My brother and I went and picked out her coffin—a beautiful one—as if somehow we could show the world how precious and wonderful Mother had been.

I planned her funeral service. The music was light and joyful to reflect Mom's love and passion for music. The message was on faith, hope, and love—mirroring Mother's philosophy of life. Her family had gathered from far and near to honour her. Our son Jim gathered up memories from various members of our family, and shared them with the church full of guests to honour mother. Then there was a tea prepared and served by the women of our church.

Always at funerals my mind goes back to the time our little son Billy died. Just as with mother, I felt like I also had gone to the very gates of heaven with Billy but

I was left behind to take up the burdens of life. It had been seven and one half months of pain and agony for Billy, as well as for Martin and me. I felt that we had said goodbye and there was no need for a funeral. I asked myself, "Why does society force a funeral upon us? Why do we have to go through another painful event? Why do we have to go to a party and face people?" I was ready to pull away. I thought of hiding in our closet, or under the branches of our huge blue spruce tree—anything to escape further pain and grief. Yet somehow as I went through all the preparations, peace seemed to settle on me. I had no tears. People were so loving and supportive. I saw and appreciated the pain in their eyes and the flowers in their hands, and I felt love. After the service I walked out to our car. In the yard of the church, I saw a dear friend. She was sobbing great sobs for the little boy whom we lost, and for our family full of grief. Though my eyes were dry at the time, I never forgot her tears or the other people who showed in various ways that they cared. From then on I appreciated funerals, and the teas that followed. Somehow they help to reconnect grief-stricken people with the world of the living while acknowledging the deep grief and pain of the loss. These lessons were very painful but I have never forgotten them.

It seems like a short time since Mother died. The good memories take prominence, while the difficult ones recede. Going back over my journals has proven this statement true. I am often surprised at how difficult it had been, I had almost forgotten. Would I do it again? Yes, a million times, yes. Mother was, and still is, so precious to me. She was not the disease, but had the disease. She remained essentially herself--loving and kind. To ease a loved one in her final years, days, and hours, is indeed a privilege. God granted me that privilege.

The final honour to my mother was to accompany her through the valley of the shadow of death

PART SEVEN

SIGNIFICANT LESSONS

1. RESPECT AND DIGNITY

It is absolutely imperative that each person with Alzheimer's disease be treated with respect and dignity. There is nothing that can replace those qualities of service. The person has a serious and vicious disease and it is not of his or her choosing. Everyone dreads, perhaps above all things, the diminishment of mental abilities. Yet it does happen, and it could happen to any one of us. If it happened to us, what we would desire is patience and understanding, which are components of respect. The Golden Rule has never lost its importance.

I hope that respect and dignity have been demonstrated by all the stories I have told. That attitude has been a personal goal of mine because I believe it so thoroughly. If we want to truly help other people, it is absolutely essential that each person be treated with dignity—children, our spouses, elderly, sick, dying, those with mental or physical disabilities—there are no exceptions. I have come to believe that it is the cry of every human heart: see me, recognize me as a person of worth, trust me, respect me, and allow me my dignity. Respect does not belittle, or diminish the person. It allows assistance when needed but in a manner that is not condescending.

2. INEFFECTIVE STRATEGIES

I have often heard comments similar to these: "She has to learn" or "How will she learn if I don't teach her?" There comes a point very early in this disease when no further learning is possible. This must be recognized and accepted by family members and other caregivers as a fact. Why persist in a useless behaviour that does more harm than good? It just reinforces the individual's belief that she is 'stupid' or 'not worth much.'

Arguing is often the outcome of trying to teach someone who is not able to learn any more, and is a senseless and degrading habit. Perhaps all family members are guilty of this at times—even me, and I know better. We hate to see the diminishment of our loved one's reasoning ability and we try to change it. Yet we can't. It is impossible.

My experience has been that the individual's perceptions, though flawed, are so strong that arguing just leads to aggression and paranoia. It is much wiser to drop the subject if possible. Try to get into the other person's perceptions, see the situation as she sees it and gently respond appropriately. Develop empathy.

3. FRIENDLINESS AND GENTLENESS

The qualities of friendliness and gentleness are vitally important. The person with Alzheimer's disease is able to detect the vibes of love, even if they are unable to verbalize. When I went to help Mom, her face would light up with a beautiful smile. Friendliness breeds friendliness, and gentleness breeds gentleness; whereas anger and impatience breed only themselves. Actually these qualities help not only the person, but they help you—they make your job much easier!

I realize that my mother's basic personality was gentle, kind, and non-aggressive and that not everyone has the same characteristics as she had. Everyone's response to this disease is unique, yet I also realize that with different treatment mother had the potential to become very aggressive. It comes back to the idea that perceptions are very important. For instance, if a person believes someone is going to mistreat, abuse, or even kill him, would it not be only human to fight back—to take any means to survive?

4. PHYSICAL HEALTH

The physical health of your loved one is very important. Ensure that he/she receives a thorough assessment for mental and physical functioning, and that there are careful follow-ups by a physician. The physician should be patient, caring, and kind, yet treat the person with dignity and respect. In addition to a good doctor, my second line of help was a caring pharmacist. Pharmacists have a great deal of knowledge about drugs and their possible interactions. Poor physical health intensifies the dementia.

You must also look after your own health. It is hard to get enough rest and relaxation. With my best efforts I was constantly tired. A night out for dinner with my husband made a great difference in my outlook and patience. There is a saying that I read or heard somewhere (I have forgotten the source): "You look after you for me, and I'll look after me for you." The physical and mental health of all partners is equally important.

5. HAVE A GOAL

The goal that I defined very definitely in my conscious thoughts was TO ENHANCE EACH DAY OF MY MOTHER'S LIFE. This goal kept me very focused when caregiving became extremely difficult. Each day I asked myself how I could enhance my mom's life that day. I might do something to make her life special, or I might arrange for someone else to take her out or do something with her that she would especially enjoy. Of course, most days we did many things that enhanced her life.

Toward the end when pressures mounted I kept reminding myself, FOCUS, REFOCUS, NOW FOCUS AGAIN. This self-talk gave me the strength and courage to go on. I used a journal to write my thoughts and record my goals. On the last day of Mom's life, when the doctor came to verify death, I said to him: "This day I enhanced my mother's life. I was with her when she died." This was important to me. I had given her my all, and I had no regrets.

6. LOOK AFTER YOURSELF

Take advantage of any help that is available, including other family members. Take responsibility, but don't try to run a one-man-show. When you leave someone else in charge, give thorough instructions on daily care and routines.

It helps to talk the situation out with loving and supportive people. I have always appreciated all the support given to me by her other caregivers, family, friends, and my church. It is a gift to be surrounded by loving people.

Take a break. Your loved one may not appreciate your absence, but it is important that you do not experience burn out. Do not feel guilty about caring first for yourself. You will become a better and more supportive caregiver.

7. CONCLUDING COMMENTS

My hope is that this record of my precious mother and her vicious disease will help some other people in similar circumstances. Mom would have liked that. In the six years since her death, I hear of a great many people who are in similar situations as ours. Whether you are caring for your mother (or loved one) in your home as I did, or in a facility, you can do it if you have the will. Despite your greatest desires, it may be impossible for you to do all that I did. Accept that, and don't feel like a failure. Do what you can and do it with dedication, love, gentleness, and great respect.

My vision while writing this book has been clear and vivid. It was to encourage other people who face similar situations, to offer my understanding and empathy to them, and to minimize the effects of this vicious disease on its victims.

My greatest fear is that you will say, "Gerry is a special person, I could never do it." (I've heard that one before!) There is nothing special about me. I am a human being with the same flaws as you. Or perhaps someone may say, "It takes too much patience, and I have never had patience." I guess another motto of mine could be, "*I can do anything, if I believe I can.*" Or you may even believe that your loved one is too far into the disease for you to try. I believe it is never too late for a loving smile and a gentle touch. You may not be able to do all I did, but I'm sure you can do something. What it takes is a determination and a willingness to give your best. You have had glimpses of my human frailties—perhaps even of a little self-pity at times (I hope not); however, the rewards greatly outweigh any of the difficulties.

The thought occurs to me that there are many daughters or sons who feel a duty to care for one of their parents in a similar situation to mine. Yet they did not have the previous relationship with their parent that I had. I never fought with my Mom in my teen years or indeed in all my life—we were very close. But how is a child to do the care when they have a load of garbage from their past! Words of advice are easy. It's really only those of experience that we listen to; however, I did have some childhood-garbage to get rid of when it came to giving tender care to my dad. I suggest that you use some mental strategies. Perhaps you could visualize yourself carrying that heavy load and crossing a bridge over a deep and roaring chasm with sharp rocks arising in it. As you look over the bridge, take that load and throw it over to be destroyed in the roaring waters and sharp rocks below—never to be recovered. If you are a believer in God, hand it to him and let him do the job for you. Then go to your parent with love in your heart, and forgiveness in your mind. Let the past go and focus on the present—you see, that is what your parent is experiencing; just the here and now and you can too. Then you can receive those final gifts of love that are priceless. The past cannot be changed, but the future for you is repairable by living with love in the present.

It is helpful to see this disease as a terminal one—for it truly is that. When people deal with the sudden death of a loved one, they never have an opportunity to say Goodbye or to build up some positive memories. That is not the case with Alzheimer's; usually there is ample time to say Goodbye and to do those things that are vitally important.

There are numerous people who suffer from this vicious disease, and unfortunately many more will succumb to it in the years to come. I hope in some small way this book will alleviate suffering and distress now and in the future.

*Life is a continual classroom
where many lessons are learned
We learn that gentleness, loving kindness,
flexibility, and focus are keys to
successful care of others*

POSTSCRIPT

The following is a list of instructions and suggestions given to others who cared for my mother. The instructions were given out in the earlier stages of the disease and my book reveals other ideas for later stages. These may offer you a few additional ideas:

General:
* Always treat her with respect and dignity.
* Let her do for herself everything she is capable of doing.
* Call her by a respectful name: either Verta or Mrs. Pouncy.
* Listen to what she has to say.
* Give her eye contact.
* Talk to her, not about her, in her presence.

Health & Safety:
* Always securely take her arm or have her take yours when going outside her home. Even in her home be alert for potential injuries or falls.
* Inform Gerry if you see any adverse health concerns.
* If Gerry is not available (which would be rare) and she becomes ill, arrange to take her to see the doctor. (Information re health resources were available)
* Ensure that she takes her proper medication when under your care. (She may mislay pills or put them in her pocket. Watch her take them please. Do not give medications to her to keep, but keep them on your person until time for dispensing them.)
* Ensure that she is warm enough. She has Raynaud's disease and poor circulation, and is usually cold even on a warm day. When she is

sitting still, we usually wrap her up in blankets found on the chesterfield, love seat, or big chair.
❀ She may need to be gently directed to the washroom. She forgets directions. Transition periods between sleep and waking, and waking and sleep are particularly confusing for her. Do not take for granted that she knows you or knows where various rooms are. Sometimes she forgets what you have told her immediately after you speak—health and various other factors impact her memory.
❀ Pour warm water into washroom basin. Encourage her to wash her hands.
❀ Be familiar with her Care Book.

Grooming:
❀ Ensure that she is clean, her hair is combed, and her clothes are clean. Make any changes in a respectful way; asking rather than commanding. She likes to look good and will positively respond to suggestions.

Activities:
❀ Verta likes to go out every day. Take the initiative to take her to places she would enjoy. Some activities are preplanned and Gerry may suggest others. All her time cannot be spent going out, so activities should be planned for time at home. Some activities might be:
❀ Reading simple Bible stories or other personal interest stories to her. She has a hearing problem, so you should speak fairly loudly and distinctly, while not shouting.
❀ Looking at books with big pictures.
❀ Watching tapes on the VCR.
❀ Simple crafts: She has simple craft materials in

her bedroom—they must be simple and you must somehow involve her in them or she will lose interest.

❀ Discussing her family, family pictures, or her china painting.

❀ In the nice weather, walking or sitting outside.

❀ Sharing a cup of tea and refreshments with her.

Ingram Content Group UK Ltd.
Milton Keynes UK
UKHW010705310323
419457UK00001B/80